Chronic Fatigue Syndrome

How To Find Facts And Get Help

by

Pamela D. Jacobs

R&E Publishers, Inc. • Saratoga, CA

Copyright © 1992 by Pamela D. Jacobs. All rights reserved. Printed in the United States of America. No part of this book may be used or reproduced in any manner whatsoever without written permission except in the case of brief quotations embodied in critical articles or reviews.

For information, write:

R&E Publishers, Inc.
P.O. Box 2008, Saratoga, CA 95070

96 95 94 93 92   5 4 3 2 1

Library of Congress Cataloging in Publication Data

by Pamela D. Jacobs   **LC NO. 92-53771**
  Chronic Fatigue Syndrome: How To Find Facts And
  Get Help.   **I.S.B.N. 0-88247-951-2**

Disclaimer: This reference guide contains information for people with Chronic Fatigue and Immune Dysfunction Syndrome (CFIDS), also known as Chronic Fatigue Syndrome (CFS) or Chronic Epstein-Barr virus (CEBV). The purpose of this guide is to provide information; not to provide medical advice or to endorse any specific theories, treatments, or products. The author and publisher assume no responsibility for any treatments chosen by a reader. Consult your health care professional for medical care and for all treatment recommendations.

Front cover design by: Mike Hudson, Copymat, San Mateo
Back cover photo by: Dino's Photography, San Francisco
Typesetting by: Diane Parker, Palo Alto

Dedication

To The CFIDS Foundation in San Francisco, Jan Montgomery and Marya Grambs, The CFIDS Association, Inc., in Charlotte, North Carolina, and to CFIDS Support Groups nationwide for providing information and encouragement to thousands of individuals.

Acknowledgements

With love to my supportive parents, Sid and Annibelle, and to my brothers: Larry, Steve, and Stan. Thanks to a dear friend, Diane Conflenti, for her editorial assistance, insights, and delightful sense of humor. To Jeffry Anderson, M.D., with sincere gratitude for providing a proper diagnosis and treatment after 11 years. Special thanks to Martin Borge, D.C., Ellen Cutler, D.C., Jan Carlson, Valerie Hearn, Ph.D., William Collinge, Ph.D., and Corey Weinstein, M.D. for quality, compassionate health care. My deep appreciation to Bob Reed, my publisher, for his guidance, patience, motivation, and contribution to this book. Thanks to Frank Petrini for his words of encouragement. And warm thanks to Pat and Curran Engel, Mary Baum, Sita L. Mulligan, Ellen Raskin-Dasher, Lenka Studnicková, Liz Chickering, Kerri Dukas, Sandra Mendoza, Chris Ailes, and to members of the San Fransico CFS Support Group for their understanding and friendship.

Contents

Acknowledgements v
1. What is Chronic Fatigue Syndrome (CFS)? 1
   Other Names for CFS 2
   List of Common CFS Symptoms 2
2. Physical Impact of CFS 3
3. Ruling Out Other Illnesses Which Can Cause Fatigue 5
4. Some Tests To Rule Out Illnesses Other Than CFS 6
5. How CFS May Be Diagnosed 7
6. Possible Causes and Contributing Factors to CFS 8
   List of Possible Contributing Factors to CFS, Immune
   System Impairment, and Illness 11
7. Socio-Economic Impact of CFS 14
8. Psychological and Emotional Impact of CFS 15
   Depression and CFS 15
9. Nutritional Imbalances 17
10. Treatment Recommendations for CFS 19
    "Natural" Treatments for CFS 21
11. Creating a Healthy Lifestyle 25
12. Living with CFS 27
13. CFS Hotline Numbers 28
    The CFIDS Association Toll-Free and
    Information Lines 30
    The CFIDS Association Information Line Menu 31
14. CFS Information 32
    Organizations Providing Information on CFS Research
    and Support Groups Outside of the U.S. 32
    Medical Libraries 33
    Health Resource Centers 33
    Key Words 34
15. CFS Support Groups and Organizations 35

16. Self-Help Information and Organizations for CFS 37
    Self-Help Retreats for CFS Offered
        Throughout the U.S. 37
    How To Start Your Own Support Group 37
    Neuropsychological Information and Evaluations 38
    Actualism (a meditation and healing arts school) 38
    Health Educational Seminars (J.I.C. and the SelfCare
        Research Center) 39
    National Health Federation (San Francisco Chapter) 40
17. Nutritional Supplements – Suppliers 40
18. Medical Test Laboratories 41
    Food Allergy Laboratory 41
    Clinical Laboratories 41
19. Health Clinics and Community Services 42
20. Recommended Reading and Tapes 44
    Books on Tape – Resources 44
    CFS Audio Tape 44
    CFS Books 44
    CFS Journal 47
    CFS Newsletters 47
    CFS Video Tapes 47
    Communication Books 47
    Environmental Books 48
    Environmental Catalogs 49
    Environmental Newsletters 49
    Financial Books 50
        —Social Security Disability Benefits Information 50
    Health and Science Newsletters 51
    Health Books 51
    Health Books and Tapes – Mail Order 54
    Nutrition, Herbs, and Supplements – Books 55
    Psychology/Self-Help Books 56
21. Research Funding for CFS 58
    Appendix—Sources for General Research 60
    CFS Telephone Directory 68
    My Personal CFS Telephone Directory 70
    Order Forms 72

1. What is Chronic Fatigue Syndrome (CFS)?

The Centers for Disease Control (CDC)* defines Chronic Fatigue Syndrome as:

1) Prolonged or recurring severely debilitating, unexplained fatigue that cuts one's activity level to 50 percent or less of what it was previously, lasting six months or longer; and

2) Fatigue not due to any other organic or psychiatric disorder —such as cancer, bacterial infection, rheumatologic disorders, or clinical depression—together with eight of these symptoms:
   1. low-grade fever
   2. sore throat
   3. painful lymph nodes in the neck or underarms
   4. muscle weakness
   5. muscle pain
   6. prolonged fatigue after exercise
   7. headaches
   8. migratory joint pain (without swelling or redness)
   9. one or more of: light sensitivity, forgetfulness, irritability, confusion, difficulty thinking or concentrating, depression
   10. sleep disturbances
   11. abrupt onset of symptoms.

Or six of the above symptoms and documentation of two of the three physical criteria below:
   1. low-grade fever
   2. inflamed throat
   3. palpable or tender lymph nodes in neck or armpits.

Currently there is no definite lab test for CFS. Therefore, a diagnosis includes ruling out other illnesses.

* Public Health Service, Centers for Disease Control, Atlanta, GA 30333. Call: (404) 332-4555 for recorded information on CFS and other diseases.

Other Names for Chronic Fatigue Syndrome (CFS):

Chronic Epstein-Barr Virus (CEBV)
Chronic Fatigue and Immune Dysfunction Syndrome (CFIDS)
Chronic Mononucleosis
Fibromyalgia (FM)
Myalgic Encephalomyelitis (ME)
"Yuppie Flu"

List of Common CFS Symptoms:

- Severe fatigue
- Recurrent flu-like illness
- Chronic sore throat
- Low-grade fevers
- Muscle and joint aches
- Insomnia
- Daytime sleepiness
- Headaches/migraines
- Changes in visual acuity
- Seizures
- Numbness and tingling
- Severe dizziness
- Spaciness
- Frightening dreams
- Depression
- Anxiety/panic attacks
- Personality changes
- Mood swings
- Psychological disorders
- Ringing in ears
- Paralysis
- Muscular weakness
- Carpal Tunnel Syndrome
- Liver malfunction
- New allergies
- Candida
- Blackouts
- Light sensitivity
- Intolerance to alcohol
- Alteration of taste, smell, hearing
- Non-restorative sleep
- Decreased sex drive
- Twitching muscles
- Inability to concentrate
- Fogginess
- Memory impairment
- Spacial disorientation
- Severe premenstrual syndrome
- Weight gain/loss
- Painful, swollen lymph nodes
- Abdominal pains
- Gas
- Frequent canker sores
- Diarrhea
- Nausea
- Heart palpitations
- Night sweats
- Rashes
- Chest pains
- Shortness of breath
- Thyroid and hormonal imbalances

2. Physical Impact of Chronic Fatigue Syndrome

Chronic Fatigue Syndrome, a highly complex disorder, causes debilitating fatigue and other symptoms, including: headaches, sore throat, fever, weakness, lymph node pain, muscle and joint pains, memory loss, and difficulty in concentrating. It can affect many systems of the body, such as: the immune system, endocrine system, nervous system, and digestive system.

CFS often attacks people suddenly and could be mistaken for the flu. Yet with CFS, people do not recover in two or three weeks, but rather continue to be ill for a longer time. By definition, CFS lasts at least six months and often lasts for years;[*] although the symptoms tend to wax and wane. This serious illness may leave as many as one-third of its victims unable to work or take care of their families. People with CFS do not always look as sick as they are, so often their illness is not taken seriously.

Women, men, and children of all races, income levels, and ages are being affected by CFS, although twice as many women as men are being diagnosed. People with CFS experience symptoms which tend to be individualistic and to fluctuate in severity. For example, some people recover in a short period of time, while others remain ill for years. People may experience severe pain and are forced to stay in bed, while others have mild symptoms and may continue working. Sometimes CFS breaks out in groups of people within communities, meaning a virus may be involved which is traveling throughout the population. One's lifestyle, family background, environment, state of the immune system, general health, diet, emotional state, etc., may determine whether or not one becomes ill with CFS. Most people who live or work closely with those who have CFS do not get the disease; thus, it does not appear to be easily contagious.[**]

[*] Holmes, G.P., Kaplan, J.E., Gantz, N.M., et al. "Chronic Fatigue Syndrome: A Working Case Definition." *Annals of Internal Medicine* (1988) 108: 387.

[**] The CFIDS Foundation, San Francisco. "Chronic Fatigue Immune Dysfunction Syndrome" (1992 brochure).

Currently this illness is a provisional diagnosis to be considered by a physician, only after all other potential causes of illness have been reasonably excluded.

Chronic Fatigue Syndrome is NOT simply "chronic fatigue." Lack of sleep, insomnia, overwork, extreme depression, or stress can cause fatigue. Fatigue may be an early warning sign for other illnesses such as lupus, multiple sclerosis, thyroid or hormonal disorders. (See: Ruling Out Other Illnesses.)

The difference between chronic fatigue and Chronic Fatigue Syndrome is: CFS causes an extremely severe form of fatigue that doesn't go away for long periods of time, in combination with a number of other physical problems such as swollen lymph nodes, flu-like symptoms, fevers, and memory loss.

CFS symptoms vary and routine medical tests may not find an organic cause; therefore, people with Chronic Fatigue Syndrome often suffer rejection by physicians, family, and friends. Not being taken seriously causes confusion and adds stress. When lab tests fail to reveal organic abnormalities, a CFS patient is often referred to a psychiatrist for depression or anxiety—implying that his or her symptoms and fatigue are psychosomatic. This skepticism is sometimes more difficult to cope with than the illness itself.

Formerly called the "Yuppie Flu," CFS may cause a physically active person to experience a sudden onset of a flu-like illness that "never goes away." Thus CFS may dramatically alter one's energy and lifestyle. All segments of the population are at risk. Adults and children of all backgrounds are experiencing this illness. However, women under 45 years of age are the most susceptible, according to the Centers for Disease Control in Atlanta, Georgia.

Many questions remain unanswered about CFS. Progress has been made in diagnosing and treating the illness, providing hope for those who are ill.

3. Ruling Out Other Illnesses Which Can Cause Fatigue

There are no specific lab tests for diagnosing CFS. Before your doctor makes a diagnosis of CFS, he or she may need to rule out other illnesses or disorders which may cause fatigue. Fatigue may be related to any of the following:

Adrenal insufficiency
Adverse drug reactions
AIDS/HIV
AIDS-related complex (ARC)
Allergies
Alzheimer's disease
Anemia
Anxiety/Panic attacks
Autoimmune diseases
Bacterial infection
Cancer
Candida albicans
Cardiovascular disorders
Chemical hypersensitivity
Chronic exposure to low level electromagnetic radiation
Clinical depression
Cognitive dysfunction
Cytomegalovirus (CMV)
Degenerative disease
Dental problems
Depression
Diabetes
Endocrine disorders
Environmental Illness (EI)
Epstein-Barr Virus (EBV)
Fibromyalgia (FM)
Gastrointestinal disorders
Herpes viruses
Hodgkin's disease
Hypogammaglobulinemia
Hypoglycemia
Immunological disorders
Lethargy
Leukemia
Liver disorders
Lupus
Lyme disease
Malnutrition
Mixed Infection Syndrome (MIS)
Mononucleosis
Multiple sclerosis
Neurological disorders
Parasites
Post-polio syndrome
Psychological disorders
Pulmonary disorders
Sleep disorders
Stress
Systemic diseases
Toxicity
Tuberculosis
Veneral diseases
Viruses/Retroviruses

4. Tests to Rule Out Illnesses Other Than Chronic Fatigue Syndrome*

1. Complete Blood Count (CBC)
    CBC evaluates your general health. If you have Chronic Fatigue Syndrome, your CBC may be normal.

2. Adrenal Function Test
    This test may reveal any adrenal insufficiency. Adrenal malfunction may cause fatigue and weakness.

3. Thyroid Function Test
    A malfunctioning thyroid can cause chronic fatigue.

4. Chest X-ray
    A chest X-ray may rule out other conditions which resemble Chronic Fatigue Syndrome. If you have CFS, your chest X-ray may be normal.

5. Urinalysis
    A urine test may reveal genital or urinary tract disorders. Fatigue may be a symptom of such disorders. A urinalysis may reveal drug abuse or toxicity. A 24-hour urinalysis may rule out any nutritional imbalances or kidney malfunction.

6. Stool Tests
    Results from a stool test on Chronic Fatigue Syndrome patients may be normal. A series of stool tests may be ordered to rule out the presence of parasites.

7. Monospot
    This test indicates infectious mononucleosis; it does not indicate CFS.

* Bolles, Edmund Blair. *Learning To Live With Chronic Fatigue Syndrome.* New York: Dell Publishing, 1990, pp. 39-41.

5. How Chronic Fatigue Syndrome May Be Diagnosed

The Centers for Disease Control's case definition of CFS is recognized as "official" and has legitimized the illness. Yet CFS is still considered a provisional diagnosis since it is based on symptoms which may be produced by other diseases, and on the exclusion of those diseases. Fortunately, pioneering CFS clinicians and researchers are making great strides in identifying specific objective markers for diagnosing CFS and for assessing patient treatment response.*

As reported in *The CFIDS Chronicle*, physicians and scientists are developing an array of tests which are increasingly sensitive and specific for CFS. As the cause and mechanism of this disease become clear, so will the clinical and laboratory parameters which define the illness. Ultimately, conclusive diagnostic standards will be developed and accepted.

Many physicians, unfamiliar with CFS, have difficulty diagnosing it. Others still do not even recognize that the illness exists. As a result, people with CFS are often misdiagnosed.

A physician may take a complete medical history, including a history of any food or drug allergies, drug use, or any possible toxic exposures. He or she may do a complete physical examination before ordering lab tests. To insure a proper diagnosis of CFS, lab work may include**:

- Viral studies: EBV, CMV, HHV-6, HSV-1 & 2, Ruebella, Coxsackie, HIV
- Basic chemistry, urine, etc. (Check for nutritional imbalances, kidney or endocrine disorders, and toxicity. NIH researchers report low cortisol levels in CFS patients.)
- Nutritional and metabolic testing

---

* The CFIDS Association, Inc., "A Guide For People With CFS," (Spring 1992) pg. 155.

** Rosenbaum, M.D., Michael, and Murray Susser, M.D. *Solving the Puzzle of Chronic Fatigue Syndrome*. Tacoma, WA: Life Sciences Press, 1992, pg. 154.

- Immune dysregulation: IgG levels with subclasses, IgA, Secretory IgA, IgM, Cellular Immune Assay with NK Cells, immune complexes
- B cells and T cells (Check immune response. EBV increases B cell levels.)
- CD8 Cells (CFS patients showed abnormalities of CD8 cells, resulting in a hyperactive immune system—according to Dr. Jay Levy.)
- Spleen, liver, adrenal, and thyroid function
- Autoimmune screening (ANA)
- Stool and antibodies for candidiasis and parasites
- Bacterial cultures
- Digestive disorders and allergies
- Brain function: SPECT, BEAM, neuropsychiatric, MRI or CAT, neurotransmitters.

6. Possible Causes and Contributing Factors to Chronic Fatigue Syndrome

Chronic Fatigue Syndrome often causes people who were once healthy, productive, and active to become physically ill and exhausted—affecting every aspect of their lives. They're not imagining symptoms or just depressed, as some doctors still suggest. Are they perhaps experiencing adverse effects of toxic chemicals or other forms of pollution? Or is the culprit a virus? No one knows.

Myths and confusion have surrounded this illness, making it difficult for patients to obtain a proper diagnosis and medical care. Lack of recognition of CFS as a "legitimate" disease has slowed research. Current findings suggest that CFS is a dysfunction of the immune system. The exact nature of this dysfunction is not yet well defined, but it can generally be viewed as an unregulated, overactive, and sometimes suppressed state—which is responsible for most of the symptoms.*

---

* "A Guide For People With Chronic Fatigue Syndrome." *The CFIDS Chronicle, Journal of the Chronic Fatigue and Immune Dysfunction Syndrome.* (Spring 1992) pp. 155-156.

Similar illnesses have been known by various names throughout history. Finding an appropriate name for CFS has been difficult because of the inability to trace its cause. There were CFS outbreaks in the 1930s, 1940s, and 1950s, but doctors thought they were seeing a variant of polio.* The misdiagnoses of polio faded after introduction of the polio vaccine. Between 1934 and 1960, from Iceland to California, there were over thirty similar outbreaks. In the mid-1980s, an outbreak at Incline Village in Lake Tahoe caught the attention of Dr. Paul Cheney, an internist. Dr. Cheney and a colleague were seeing patients with debilitating exhaustion, weakness, headaches, fevers, swollen glands, poor concentration, and other symptoms—now known as classic CFS symptoms. Dr. Cheney read in a medical journal article that the Epstein-Barr virus (EBV), which causes mononucleosis, may play a role in producing chronic fatigue. Wondering if that virus was related to his fatigue cases, he took some blood tests and found that many of his patients carried unusually high amounts of the EBV antibody.

An antibody is a protein made by the immune system. Antibodies attack and destroy foreign proteins which enter the bloodstream. The presence of an antibody in the blood usually indicates an active viral infection.

Dr. Cheney's findings suggested that he might have found a new infectious disease threatening to become a national epidemic. Several researchers were interested in Dr. Cheney's findings, including Dr. Anthony Komaroff, of the Harvard Medical School. Dr. Komaroff began working with Dr. Cheney; and to this day, Dr. Komaroff is one of the leading practitioners who study CFS. He developed an active treatment program for CFS patients, following their progress to track the course of the disease.

The Centers for Disease Control (CDC) in Atlanta, Georgia responded to Dr. Cheney's clinical implications. Involved in tracking epidemics and mass poisonings to determine their sources, the CDC sometimes imposes strict emergency health

---

* Bolles, Edmund Blair. *Learning To Live With Chronic Fatigue Syndrome*. New York: Dell Publishing, 1990, pp. 8-9.

regulations on communities. CDC doctors work as medical detectives, searching to find the source of an epidemic.

In 1985, the CDC sent Dr. Jonathan Kaplan and Dr. Gary Holmes, to Lake Tahoe to look into Dr. Cheney's findings suggesting that EBV was a new viral epidemic. However, the investigators reported that they could not be sure that the EBV was involved in the outbreak. A few years later, Drs. Kaplan and Holmes helped to establish a diagnostic criteria for the disease, but it does not explain the cause of CFS.

In 1985, the Portland *Oregonian* printed an article, "Is This You?"—describing classic CFS symptoms. Those who respónded formed the first support group for people with Chronic Fatigue Syndrome. A national network now exits which provides help and information to patients, doctors, and the general public. (See: CFS Support Groups and Organizations.)

One CFS researcher, Jay A. Levy, M.D., Professor of Medicine and Research Associate at the University of California, San Francisco, states: "This complex disorder is a physical ailment, not a psychological one as was once believed. CFS impairs the body's immune system; both CFS and AIDS degenerate the immune system, but CFS is not AIDS. With CFS, the immune system may get stuck in overdrive, trying to rid the body of infection. With AIDS, the immune system can shut down drastically."

Dr. Levy and Dr. Carol Jessop, a California internist, and their colleagues have been trying to isolate specific markers in their CFS patients. So far, their studies have isolated three markers for this illness detectable through blood tests.

Dr. Levy believes that CFS is not contagious, as some may think. Clusters of CFS appearing within families or communities, may be due to "simultaneous exposure to the causative agent."

Dr. Jessop has seen over eleven hundred CFS patients. At a symposium on CFS, she reported a recovery rate of 88 percent—59 percent of whom fully regained their previous health. She says, "I have an interest in women's health areas, particularly those that are dubbed 'controversial' diseases and to me clearly have an etiology [a physical cause]...." She sees a number of male patients; however, 83 percent of her CFS patients are women.

Dr. Jessop believes that *Candida albicans*, a common yeast, is producing a neurotoxin called d-arabinol, which may cause CFS symptoms. While the neurotoxin is not lethal, it may cause debilitation. If Dr. Jessop's theory is correct, it is a gross understatement to call CFS's primary symptom "fatigue." She believes that "contemporary lifestyles have changed the body's ecosystem." While this "yeast theory" is not new, hundreds of people have recovered following Dr. Jessop's treatment program.

The "yeast theory" was first developed by Dr. C. Orian Truss, an allergist in Birmingham, Alabama. Another allergist in Tennessee, Dr. William Crook, elaborates on this subject in his book, *Chronic Fatigue Syndrome and The Yeast Connection*. The theory, however, remains controversial.

Dr. Tom Wu, of the SelfCare Research Center in Belmont, California, has helped several people with CFS by treating candida-overgrowth. He recommends: 1) dietary changes (limit: sugar, dairy products, alcohol, caffeine, fruit juices); 2) a cleansing program; 3) light exercise; and 4) taking appropriate supplements.

List of Possible Contributing Factors to CFS, Immune System Impairment, and Illness:

- Overuse of drugs, such as antibiotics or alcohol, long-term use of birth control pills, cigarette smoking, or second-hand smoke.
- Candida over-growth caused by use of antibiotics, birth control pills, or improper diet. (Recommended reading: *Lick the Sugar Habit* by Dr. Nancy Appleton, and *Chronic Fatigue Syndrome and The Yeast Connection* by Dr. William Crook.)
- Transference of illnesses, viruses, and bacteria from animals to previously uninfected human populations. (As described in Paul and Anne Ehrlich's *The Population Explosion*. New York: Touchstone, 1990, pg. 149.)

- Polio vaccines, made from green monkey parts, may have mutated in our bodies—causing immune system disorders. (Well documented by Dr. Eve Snead, c/o Wellness Council, 126 E. Ridgewood, San Antonio, TX 78212.)
- Transference of illnesses, viruses, and bacteria in hospitals.
- Viruses, including Herpes: HSV-1, HSV-2, HHV6, CEBV (causes mononucleosis), CMV, Varicella-zoster virus (chicken pox, shingles), Rubella, influenza; retroviruses, such as Human T-Cell Leukemia—HTLV 2 or spumavirus; or a reaction to viruses being in the body for an extended time.
- Bacterial infections.
- Family background.
- Sexually transmitted diseases.
- Heavy metal poisoning, such as lead, mercury, cadmium, or aluminum.
- Dental problems: including mercury fillings which may cause CFS in some people. (In their book, *Solving the Puzzle of Chronic Fatigue Syndrome*, Drs. Rosenbaum and Susser write: "Mercury invades the central nervous system, causing neurologic dysfunction. It also invades the kidneys and other organ systems...They suspect that many patients with CFS have too much mercury in their body. Some dentists remove the amalgam from patients with evidence of mercury toxicity causing fatigue." Removing the amalgam may correct chronic fatigue. For more information, read *It's All In Your Head* by Hal Huggins, D.D.S.)
- Poor diet, anemia, eating disorders, digestive problems, and malnutrition. (A diet of too much fat, sugar, and protein may weaken the immune system.)
- Food additives, preservatives, saccharin, aspartame, caffeine, or MSG. (In his book, *In Bad Taste: The MSG Syndrome*, George R. Schwartz, M.D. describes how living without monosodium glutamate can reduce headache, depression and asthma. [New York: A Signet Book, 1988.] In *Lick the Sugar Habit*, Dr. Nancy Appleton describes how saccharin, aspartame, caffeine, etc. affect health and well-being.)
- Silicon implants (in some cases).
- Stress, emotional problems, depression, anxiety, post traumatic stress disorder (PTSD).

- Environmental pollution such as toxic waste, oil spills, global warming, SMOG, acid rain, fires, volcanic eruptions, nuclear disasters and waste. (In March 1992, CNN reported that the U.S. army sprayed a toxic chemical throughout the San Francisco Bay Area in California—and in other states—as an "experiment" in the early 1950s. The government did not warn citizens about it. CNN confirmed that this chemical sprayed over many residential areas was "definitely toxic.")
- Over-population. (In *The Population Explosion*, Paul and Anne Ehrlich write that "From global warming to rainforest destruction, famine, and air and water pollution—over-population stands out as our number-one environmental problem.")
- The hole in the ozone layer. (In spring 1992, NASA scientists studied the thinning of the ozone. They reported that "Without the ozone layer to shield Earth's surface from ultra-violet rays, humans can suffer a dangerous increase in skin cancers, eye cataracts, and damage to the immune system...." [Perlman, David. "Scientists Discover Huge Increase in Threat to Ozone. NASA research focused on Arctic Circle," *San Francisco Chronicle*. February 1992.].)
- Pesticide spraying. (Malathion used to kill Medflies may be harmful to humans, yet its use continues. [Associated Press. "Doctors May Oppose Medfly Spraying. Vote set today on California Medical Association resolution." March 1990.].)
- Sick Building Syndrome (indoor air pollution from toxins, paint, cleaning materials, improper ventilation, chemicals, plastics, formaldehyde.)
- Radiation and electromagnetic fields—such as computer monitors, televisions, microwaves, power lines. Radiation from high altitude when flying.
- Allergies caused by pollens, pollution, foods (such as dairy products).
- Hormones in dairy products.
- Exposure to toxins, pesticides, parasites in foods and water.
- Travel exposes one to foreign viruses or bacteria.
- Breathing stale, germ-filled, recycled air while flying. (Schmitz, Anthony. "Who Took The Air Out of Airplanes? And Other Sickening Mysteries of Flying." *Health*. February/

March 1992, pp. 63-65.) (For example, in 1985, on a flight from Amsterdam to Los Angeles, many passengers became very ill with influenza. Several people almost died. The Health Department in Los Angeles contacted passengers to study the problem. Perhaps if all passengers paid a few dollars extra per flight, the airlines could afford to recycle fresh air into their planes.)

Note: To improve health, begin making lifestyle changes. For example, limit exposure to toxins, avoid second-hand smoke, and eat healthy foods.

7. Socio-Economic Impact of Chronic Fatigue Syndrome

Any chronic illness can cause financial problems and CFS is no exception. Often people with CFS experience drastic lifestyle changes. They may spend thousands of dollars searching for a diagnosis and trying various treatments. They may be unable to continue working because of low or fluctuating energy levels. Some may be unable to qualify for financial aid, disability benefits, or health insurance because CFS is not recognized as a legitimate disease in many areas. This dilemma places them in a serious financial bind, causing emotional stress and jeopardizing well-being. Some people with CFS are able to work on a part-time, flexible schedule at home.

Along with financial problems, one's family and social life may be seriously affected by CFS. Chronic Fatigue Syndrome can make or break any close relationship because some lifestyle change is inevitable with any chronic illness. One's family is usually the primary source of support for a person with CFS. This illness may cause one to need more, while giving less which may cause feelings of guilt or helplessness. It is beneficial for people with CFS and their families to get emotional support and to maintain open, honest communication. With low energy and other CFS symptoms, it is often difficult for one to keep up socially with a spouse, children, friends, or colleagues. Many people with CFS report an inability to keep commitments because of fluctuating energy levels and other symptoms. Therefore, it is vital to pace oneself, to set up healthy limits, and to arrange a flexible schedule whenever possible, based upon how one is feeling. Clear communication about one's needs helps others to understand. Also it may prevent others from feeling rejected or "stood up" if plans must be changed.

Solutions must be found for coping with this challenging illness when one lives alone. Organizations, such as the Center for Independent Living, may be able to provide help and support. (See: CFS Hotline Numbers.)

8. Psychological and Emotional Impact of Chronic Fatigue Syndrome

People with CFS may experience psychological or emotional symptoms such as denial, anger, fear, anxiety, depression, mood swings, frustration, mourning, hopelessness, loss of personal control, or devastation. Those who accept the fact that they have a chronic illness and adjust to it generally cope better than those who deny CFS. To overcome the sense of isolation, they may join support groups and help each other. Understanding, hope, and optimism help with healing and recovery. (See: Self-Help and Support Groups for CFS.)

Depression and Chronic Fatigue Syndrome

Many doctors still insist that CFS is caused by depression because symptoms of depression mimic some CFS symptoms. However, CFS involves a number of physical symptoms—such as fevers, swollen glands, memory loss, muscle weakness and joint pain—which are not caused by depression. People with clinical depression tend to lose interest in their daily activities, while people with CFS generally remain interested in their activities; although in severe stages they may often lack the energy to carry out those activities. One may have depression in addition to other illnesses, including CFS. The illnesses are not mutually exclusive.

According to Dr. Valerie Hearn, a psychologist in San Francisco, "There is much evidence that one's state of mind can greatly influence one's physical wellness or illness, and vice versa. CFS has many symptoms in common with two classes of psychological difficulties—those involving depression and anxiety. Among symptoms that CFS has in common with depressive disorders are: fatigue, short-term memory loss, confusion, irritability, difficulty thinking or concentrating, sleep disturbances, weight loss or gain, and decreased sex drive. Symptoms in common with anxiety difficulties include: shortness of breath, nightsweats, diarrhea, dizziness, chest pains, numbness, tingling, and panic attacks."

Dr. Hearn believes that, "CFS patients are often unable to do many things that formerly contributed to their psychological sense of well-being. The many losses associated with a forced reduction in activity can cause depression and anxiety, or exacerbate psychological difficulties which already exist. Because there is such a close connection between mind and body it could be useful for a person with CFS to consult with a psychologist who specializes in the treatment of depression and anxiety, and one who is educated about CFS, in order to speed healing. Some people may find self-help groups beneficial for dealing with relationship and health problems."

Dr. Jerome Marmorstein, Assistant Clinical Professor of Medicine, University of Southern California, practices Internal Medicine in Santa Barbara, California. He and Nanette Marmorstein co-wrote *Awakening from Depression.**

Dr. Marmorstein has developed a program for depression and anxiety that is "safe, simple, inexpensive; and it is often more effective than drug therapy. It promotes an increase in alertness and energy, rather than sedation and drowsiness." His "Four Metabolic Steps" to help with fatigue, anxiety and depression are: 1) avoiding all caffeine; 2) limiting intake of sweets and refined sugars (but not fresh fruits); 3) limiting the

---

* Jerome Marmorstein, M.D., and Nanette Marmorstein. *Awakening from Depression: A Mind/Body Approach to Emotional Recovery.* Santa Barbara, CA: Woodbridge Press Publishing Company, 1992, pg. 15.

use of alcohol; and 4) getting regular exercise—as little as a 20-minute walk daily. He believes this regimen helps because "it affects the metabolism of several adrenalin-type hormones called biogenic amines, whose imbalance in the brain has been implicated in anxiety and depression." He suggests exercise for improvement in energy, anxiety, depression, and sense of well-being—both physically and emotionally. Exercise need not be vigorous but should be regular. (Consult a physician before beginning an exercise program. CFS patients should not over-exercise.)

Lifting depression is a step-by-step process. Learning self-care skills helps many people to feel better and to feel more in control. For others, a professional may recommend a combination of therapy, medication, and other steps toward recovery. Depression is one of the most treatable mood disorders known, once a treatment plan is begun.* Therapy sheds light on self-defeating behavior and problems in relationships. There are over 200 different kinds of therapy to teach people new coping skills and to help raise self-esteem. Help is just a phone call away. (See: CFS Hotline Numbers.)

9. Nutritional Imbalances

Meeting one's nutritional needs is essential for optimum health. Studies have shown how imbalances of certain vitamins and minerals can cause physical, mental, and emotional health problems. People with Chronic Fatigue Syndrome may benefit by having a nutritional evaluation to rule out any imbalances. (Consult with your doctor before taking supplements.)

In *Nutrition Concepts and Controversies* (New York: West Publishing Company, 1991), Hamilton, Whitney, and Sizer write: "Depressed mood is linked to eating behavior and time of day. Hunger, lack of sleep, and over-work can cause depression and poor performance. Depression can disturb both diet and

---

* Health Education Center, Kaiser Permanente Medical Center. "Overcoming Depression: Opening the Window to Recovery." Krames Communications, 1987.

sleep patterns. A type of depression, known as major depression, affects the appetite and causes weight loss. Another connection of eating behavior with depression is called Seasonal Affective Disorder (SAD). Most people with SAD have increased appetites, mostly for carbohydrate."

The authors discuss the relationship between vitamins, trace minerals, and the brain: "Energy-yielding nutrients, particularly carbohydrate and protein, affect neurotransmitter synthesis and mood. However, in the synthesis of neurotransmitters—whether norepinephrine, dopamine, or serotonin—other nutrients are involved. Iron is needed in one of the first steps. Vitamin B6 and riboflavin are needed in the later steps." These nutrients are only three among many which may affect mental state if a decificiency occurs. Some nutritional deficiencies can cause anemia and mental symptoms...." Other deficiencies which may affect health are:

- Protein-energy deficiency may cause apathy, fretfulness, lack of energy, and poor appetite.
- Thiamin deficiency may cause confusion, uncoordinated movements, depressed appetite, irritability, insomnia, fatigue, personality changes, or depression.
- Riboflavin deficiency may cause depression, hysteria, psychopathic behavior, or lethargy.
- Niacin deficiency may cause irritability, agitated depression, headaches, sleeplessness, memory loss, emotional instability, or mental confusion.
- Vitamin B6 deficiency can cause irritability, insomnia, weakness, depression, abnormal brainwave patterns, convulsions, the mental symptoms of anemia, fatigue, or headaches.
- Folacin deficiency can cause the mental symptoms of anemia, tiredness, apathy, weakness, forgetfulness, mild depression, abnormal nerve function, irritability, headache, disorientation, confusion, or inability to perform simple calculations.
- Vitamin B12 deficiency may cause degeneration of the peripheral nervous system and anemia.

- Vitamin C deficiency may cause hysteria, depression, listlessness, lassitude, weakness, social introversion, possible anemia, and fatigue.
- Vitamin A deficiency can result in anemia.
- Iron deficiency may cause fatigue, weakness, headaches, pallor, listlessness, irritability, and the mental symptoms of anemia.
- Magnesium deficiency can cause apathy, personality changes, and hyper-irritability.
- Copper deficiency can cause iron-deficiency anemia.
- Zinc deficiency may lead to poor appetite, failure to grow, iron-deficiency anemia, irritability, emotional disorders, and mental lethargy.

Nutrients affect brain function in many other ways. But this list shows how dramatically the way people eat can affect their physical, mental, and emotional health.

10. Treatment Recommendations for Chronic Fatigue Syndrome

Currently there is no known cure for CFS. According to Dr. Michael Rosenbaum and Dr. Murray Susser, co-authors of *Solving the Puzzle of Chronic Fatigue Syndrome*, "Our approach is to maintain an aggressive and sustained attack directed at each of the multiple causes of this complex disease. The range of treatments for CFS stretches from zero to infinity. Unfortunately for many patients with CFS the conventional approach usually hangs near the zero end of our continuum.... In recent years, the tendency toward treating CFS has been to recommend antidepressants or the use of histamine-2-blockers.... Patients may try anything and everything from standard medicine to 'crystal power.' The old adage that the understanding of a disease is inversely proportional to the number of treatments, certainly applies here. Because there is no simple cure, there are many recommendations."

Dr. Rosenbaum and Dr. Susser* suggest a four-step CFS treatment program:

1) *Treat mixed infections.*
    Medical history, physical exam, and lab tests to rule out illnesses.
    Treat over-growth of candida or parasites with medication or herbs.

2) *Treat mixed conditions.*
    Treat infections such as allergies, anemia, toxicity, thyroid and adrenal gland insufficiencies.

3) *Treat the core CFS viruses.*
    Neutralize viruses.
    Stimulate the immune response.

4) *Heal the nervous system.*
    Enhance energy, mental alertness, and cognition.
    Alleviate depression, anxiety, insomnia, and pain.

Doctors have found that the most successful treatment for Chronic Fatigue Syndrome combines extensive rest, easing of individual symptoms, providing emotional support, and helping with adaptation to the challenges of a chronic condition. Improving diet and maintaining a positive mental attitude are also beneficial.

The *CFIDS Treatment News*, published by The CFIDS Foundation in San Francisco, recommends that you:
- Find a doctor or nurse who knows about CFS, knows how to diagnose and treat it, and is willing to work with you over time.
- Educate yourself about the illness because there are many myths about CFS and you will need to know the facts.
- Educate your friends and family about the serious nature of your illness, so that they may help you to cope with the disease and the changes it has brought about in your life.

---

* Rosenbaum, M.D., Michael, and Susser, M.D., Murray, *Solving the Puzzle of Chronic Fatigue Syndrome*. Tacoma, WA: Life Sciences Press, 1992.

- Get plenty of rest. Do not push yourself beyond your limits.
- Do light to moderate exercise. Avoid strenuous exercise which can make the symptoms worse.
- Join a support group to help with making any necessary life changes and to reduce the isolation which CFS can create.
- Consider seeing a counselor or therapist as depression is a major, debilitating, and sometimes life-threatening symptom of the disease.

"Natural" Treatments for Chronic Fatigue Syndrome

"Natural" treatments are also recommended for CFS patients by some doctors. (Consult your own physician before beginning any type of treatment program.) "The term 'natural medicine' refers to those techniques and skills, or adjustments in living habits which aid and encourage the individual to reach a better state of health through internal healing mechanisms. All biological systems have the capacity for self-organization and renewal. The human body has an inherent power to heal itself. Natural therapies try to stimulate the body/mind's internal mechanisms to restore healthy structure and function."*

Some forms of natural healing which may be beneficial for CFS, include:
- Acupuncture and Acupressure (Oriental healing methods)
- Biofeedback (A stress reduction technique)
- Chi Gung/Qi Gong (Chinese energy enhancing movements/ techniques)
- Chiropractic (Spinal and joint alignment)
- Craniosacral therapy (Cerebral spinal fluid flow enhancement)
- Exercise (Light to moderate exercise for physical and mental well-being)

---

* Weinstein, M.D., Corey. "What is Natural Medicine?" (This brochure is currently out of print. For more information, write: 4827 Geary Blvd., San Francisco, CA 94118.)

- Herbal therapy (Consult your doctor before taking herbs)
- Homeopathy* (See footnote for explanation)
- Hydrotherapy (For relaxation and healing)
- Hypnotherapy (For stress reduction)
- Massage and bodywork (Relaxes muscles and body, improves circulation)
- Meditation and relaxation techniques
- Nutritional therapy (Consult your doctor before taking supplements)
- Osteopathic manipulation (For mobilizing joints to improve circulation)
- Psychic and spiritual healing
- Reflexology (Massaging pressure points in the hands and feet for healing)
- Tai Chi (Chinese exercises for increased energy flow)
- Therapeutic fasting and cleansing diet therapy (Consult your doctor)
- Visualization and affirmations for healing
- Yoga (Postures for stretching, strengthening, and rejuvenating the body).

---

* Homeopathic practitioners treat patients by using minute, non-toxic doses of plant, mineral, or animal substances. Specific medicines are chosen based upon the "law of similar;" that is, a substance which creates a specific set of symptoms in a healthy person when given in toxic dose will cure these "similar" symptoms in a sick person when given in specially prepared doses. Since symptoms are the body's efforts to deal with stress and to defend/heal itself, homeopathic medicines work with, rather than against, a person's overall defense system—providing a gentle but powerful healing stimulus. "Discover Homeopathy." Homeopathic Educational Services, 2124 Kittredge Street, Berkeley, CA 94704. Call: 800-359-9051 for information, books, tapes.

Because natural medicine depends on the person's own healing effort, great attention is placed on self-care. Proper food, rest, fresh air, and appropriate exercise are as important as any medicine, herb, or treatment. Natural treatment implies respect for the human body and its ways of overcoming illness. Many people find that by understanding their own rhythms and healing processes, they are more able to give themselves time and support required for a healing effort.*

Natural and standard medicines have different perspectives and approaches:

	Natural Medicine	Standard Medicine
Illness	– is an individual expression of imbalance	– occurs in well-defined groups based on pathology
Symptoms	– are evidence of disharmony and one's attempt to restore order – are analyzed to follow the progress of treatment	– are bad – successful treatment makes them go away
Diagnosis	– the understanding of the phenomenon of the illness – the whole person is taken into account	– the search for the structural cause
Treatment	– individualized and based on the entire expression of the disorder – self-care (what the client does) is emphasized.	– based on the pathologic diagnosis – what the doctor does is emphasized.

© 1985 Corey Weinstein, M.D.

* Weinstein, M.D., Corey. "What is Natural Medicine?" (This brochure is currently out of print. For more information, write: 4827 Geary Blvd., San Francisco, CA 94118.)

People with CFS must identify their limits and operate within them. Symptoms tend to be aggravated by stress and improved by rest. Some CFS doctors suggest meditation, yoga, developing a positive attitude, healthy lifestyle changes, emotional support, proper nutrition, and giving up smoking and alcohol. Vitamin and mineral supplements, especially vitamin B-complex, vitamin C, magnesium, trace minerals, and herbs may build strength and boost the immune system. Algae supplements containing essential amino acids are recommended by some doctors for CFS.

Dr. Ellen Cutler, of the Cutler Chiropractic Clinic in Larkspur, California, has helped a number of people with CFS by "utilizing chiropractic adjustments to relieve any chronic nerve irritation which stresses the body, and by treating any digestive disorders with plant enzymes to strengthen the immune system." She says, "It is important to use both treatments to bring the body back to homeostasis. Plant enzymes aid in the body's digestion, assimilation, and utilization of food nutrients. They may also help to clear up intestinal toxemia, a common cause of many disorders and diseases. Intestinal toxemia results from a certain type of diet or from intestinal obstruction. Proper diet and elimination, along with exercise are beneficial."

When a person with CFS has an increase in energy, he or she may do light stretching exercises to tone muscles. Some exercises may be done in bed while reclining, such as leg lifts and arm stretches. Television shows, such as "Sit and Be Fit," or non-impact exercise videos, are highly motivational.

CFS symptoms tend to wax and wane; therefore, a person may go from needing bedrest to being able to function almost normally. This fluctuation of energy can make it difficult to plan ahead, to make commitments, or to hold a job. Still, one can take advantage of times of increased energy, being careful not to overdo it—a common pitfall. Pacing oneself is essential. Massage, physical therapy, adequate rest, proper diet, light exercise, and support from family and friends will help to create a healthier, happier life.

11. Creating a Healthy Lifestyle

William Collinge, Ph.D., of Self-Help Retreats in Sebastopol, California, suggests taking a "Lifestyle Self-Assessment" and making positive changes to activate the healer within. He recommends following these healthy guidelines and affirmations:

1. *Nutrition.*
   I drink plenty of purified water and I eat fresh fruits and vegetables. I eat healthy foods on a regular schedule. I take appropriate nutritional supplements (according to my doctor's advice). I avoid refined sugar; minimize red meat intake; and avoid alcohol and caffeine. I read labels on food packages and limit processed foods.

2. *Habits.*
   I avoid breathing smoke. I limit watching television.

3. *Environment.*
   My environment is free of toxic chemicals and fumes. I create an environment which is relatively quiet, peaceful, beautiful, and uplifting.

4. *Relationships.*
   I communicate my feelings, wants, and needs clearly. I say "no" without guilt. I am free of unresolved conflicts and free of past hurts. I avoid "toxic" relationships. I have relationships which nourish me.

5. *Emotional expression.*
   I allow and express sadness and I cry freely. I allow and express fear, anger, love, joy, etc. I laugh freely and I smile often.

6. *Self-esteem.*
   I am free of guilt and self-judgment. I forgive myself for past mistakes. I love and accept myself, unconditionally.

7. *Alone time.*
   I spend some quality time alone each day. I let my mind rest. I relax. I spend time in introspection and meditation.

8. *Activity.*
   I get mild, comfortable exercise when I feel able. My work activity is free of anxiety and compulsiveness. My homemaking activity is free of anxiety and compulsiveness. I allow myself to rest whenever I need to.

9. *Pleasure and enjoyment.*
   I get some pleasure each day. I spend time with nurturing friends.

10. *Purpose in life.*
    I have personal goals which make my life worthwhile. I have a deep, valuable purpose for getting well. I truly believe in my purpose for getting well. I am living life according to my deeper values.

11. *Physical touch and contact with others.*
    I have physical contact with others. I give and receive affection.

12. *The spiritual dimension of life.*
    I have a spiritual or religious understanding for my life which assists me to feel peaceful, hopeful, and at ease with my life.

13. *Self-Help.*
    I actively seek information about my health on my own. I ask my doctor questions and keep asking until I am satisfied. I practice some form of self-help activity each day.

For people with CFS, Dr. Collinge recommends using his "50% solution" for awareness and management of daily energy level:

1. I appraise how much energy I have today.

2. I only expend 50% of it—keeping the other 50% for myself. Like money in a savings account, I keep energy in reserve to heal my body. This helps to guard against the tendency to over-do activites on my better days which could trigger a relapse.

12. Living with Chronic Fatigue Syndrome

Chronic Fatigue Syndrome is not terminal, although some patients have difficulty coping with the many losses and challenges associated with this illness. Besides health problems, one may experience loss of income, career, self-esteem, friendships, marriage, home, car, lifestyle, etc. A doctor with CFS said, "There's nothing CFS can not take away from you." However, one must not lose hope.

In any healing process, belief in one's recovery is vital. Following is a list of suggestions to facilitate mental, physical, and emotional well-being:

- Create new priorities in your life
    - Daily health care is priority number one
- Come out of "denial" about CFS, accept it and deal with it directly
- Maintain a positive attitude and a sense of humor
- Set appropriate limits with yourself and others
- Be true to yourself
- Develop and maintain healthy, honest communication
- Listen to your body, and pace yourself according to your body's needs
- Nurture your self-esteem and self-love
- Do yoga and meditation, go for walks, breathe fresh air
- Listen to your favorite music and sing along.

CFS forces one to re-evaluate life, to let go of unhealthy habits, to create a healthier lifestyle, and to get "back to basics." This process can be a positive experience—a "spring cleaning" of sorts. People with CFS often benefit by renewed spirituality. Laughter uplifts the spirit, and studies show that it also boosts the immune system (according to Dr. Robert Ornstein and Dr. David Sobel in *Healthy Pleasures*). Expressing inner feelings—such as disappointment, sadness, or anger—helps one to cope with depression and to deal with losses. A person with CFS needs understanding, acceptance, and kindness. Family, friends, and even pets can boost morale with love and affection.

Along with proper medical care and financial assistance, therapy can provide a stable foundation for recovery. But treatment and therapy can be very expensive when one is chronically ill and unable to work. County mental health centers, clinics, and nationwide CFS Support Groups offer help and information. Organizations, such as The CFIDS Foundation in San Francisco, provide referrals to doctors, therapists, and support groups. Whenever possible, please support their on-going research and efforts. (See: CFS Support Groups and Organizations, Health Resources, Hotline Numbers, and Research Funding.)

13. Chronic Fatigue Syndrome Hotline Numbers

For information on treatments, coping with CFS, names of doctors, etc., contact:

Centers for Disease Control
Call for recorded information on CFS and other diseases: **(404) 332-4555**

The CFIDS Association, Inc.
P. O. Box 220398
Charlotte, N.C. 28222
Toll-Free: (800) 44-CFIDS
Recorded information: (900) 988-CFID
($2 for first minute and $1 for each minute thereafter)

The CFIDS Foundation
965 Mission Street, Suite 425
San Francisco, CA 94103
(415) 882-9986
Hours: Mon, Tues, Wed, Thurs 1-3 pm Pacific Standard Time. Daily telephone counseling and referrals to knowledgeable physicians, support groups, disability lawyers, and other resources. The Foundation trains/educates health care professionals, volunteers, and the general public. Call for appointment. Physicians' packets are free to doctors; and available to patients at $10 each. Patients' packets are free and provide general information about CFS.

Center for Medical Consumers
(Reference library available on walk-in basis only)
237 Thompson Street
New York, N.Y. 10012
(212) 674-7105

Massachusetts CFIDS Association
808 Main Street
Waltham, Mass 02154
(617) 893-4415

National CFS Association
3521 Broadway, Suite 222
Kansas City, MO 64111
(816) 931-4777
Note: For information packet about CFS groups send $1 for postage and handling.

The Lung Line is a toll free number established by the National Jewish Center for Immunology and Respiratory Medicine in Denver, Colorado, to answer questions about CFS. Call: **(800) 222-5864 (LUNG)**. Hours: M-F, 8am-5 pm, Mountain Time.

24-hour information hotline by the **Indiana CFS Support Group: (317) 352-9191**

Greater San Francisco Bay Area CFS Support Group: (510) 284-CARE

Crisis Hotline for the Disabled: 1 (800) 426-4263.

Call the Yellow Pages' **Suicide Prevention** Counselors or **911** to prevent suicide. Call mental health agencies for information, support, and referrals to therapists.

The CFIDS Association's Toll-Free and Information Lines

For timely, accurate information on CFS by experts in the field, The CFIDS Association has two hotline numbers:

Toll-Free: (800) 44-CFIDS

The Toll-Free Line uses the "voice mail" system. By pressing one number on your telephone, your call can be directed to the appropriate "mailbox," whether you're a first time caller, health care professional, current member, or with the media. By leaving your name and address, The CFIDS Association will respond to your request for more information on CFS and their membership services.

900 Number for Recorded Information: (900) 988-CFID

($2 for first minute and $1 for each minute thereafter)

The caller is given a brief introduction to the system and informed of the charges. A list of general topics is then provided. The caller chooses a general topic, at which time a listing of sub-topics is provided. The caller may listen to any of the topics/subtopics, then return to the main menu at any time, simply by hitting the star (*) key. Charges for each call placed will appear on the caller's monthly telephone bill. (See: The CFIDS Information Line Menu.)

Note: Health care professionals wishing to contribute to information may call: (800) 44-CFIDS. Leave your name, topic, and phone number in the health care mailbox.

For contributions to research and efforts to disseminate information, call the 900 number.

Disclaimer: The information has been reviewed by the CFIDS medical consultant, Dr. Charles Lapp. However, each recording represents only the views of the individual presenting the topic. The CFIDS Association and the Information Line do not dispense medical advice, nor do they endorse any specific medical hypothesis or product. They assume no responsibility for any treatment undertaken by a caller.

The CFIDS Association Information Line Menu

For recorded information about Chronic Fatigue Syndrome: Call: (900) 988-CFID—$2 for first minute and $1 for each minute thereafter.

Main Menu:

- Overview of CFIDS
    What is CFIDS?
    What causes CFIDS?
    How is CFIDS diagnosed?
    What are the symptoms?
    Is CFIDS contagious?

- The CFIDS Association
    Description, objectives, and goals
    The CFIDS Chronicle Library

- Treatment
    Treatment overview
    Kutapressin
    Ampligen
    Ampligen – a patient's perspective
    Various treatments

- Diagnosis
    Diagnostic overview
    Symptom diagnosis
    Laboratory diagnosis
    Concentration/memory loss

- Research Updates
    Various reports, as available

- CACTUS
    Overview and how to join
    CDC and NIH updates
    Washington updates

- Alternative Treatments
    National CFIDS Buyers Club
    Coenzyme Q10
    Super LEM

- CFIDS-Related Health Issues
    Endometriosis
    Fibromyalgia
    Yeast infections

- CFIDS in Children
    Overview
    Treatment

14. Chronic Fatigue Syndrome Information

The Centers for Disease Control and the National Institutes of Health send free CFS information packets upon request.

Centers for Disease Control
Attn. Josephine Lister
Building 6, Room 121
Atlanta, Georgia 30333
(404) 639-1338

National Institute of Allergy and Infectious Diseases
Office of Communications
Building 31, Room 7A - 32
Bethesda, Maryland 20892

Organizations Providing Information on CFS Research and Support Groups Outside of the United States

A.N.Z.M.E. Society
P. O. Box 35-429, Browns Bay
Aukland 10, New Zealand

Myalgic Encephalomyelitis Association
P. O. Box 8
Stanford le Hope 8 EL
Essex SS17 8EX England

Medical Libraries

For current medical information, contact a medical library in your area—such as this one in San Francisco:

University of California, San Francisco – Library
530 Parnasus Avenue
San Francisco, CA 94122
(415) 476-2334

This medical library is open to the public. It has a medical database, journals and books. However, one needs a library card to check out books.

Days:	Hours:
Monday – Friday	8 am to 11 pm
Saturday	9 am to 6 pm
Sunday	Noon to 9 pm

Health Resource Centers

Contact health resource centers, such as Planetree in San Francisco, a health information service, library, and bookstore.

Planetree Health Resource Center at California Pacific Medical Center
2040 Webster Street
San Francisco, CA 94115
Phone: **(415) 923-3680**

Open to the Public:

Days:	Hours:
Tuesday – Friday:	11 am–5 pm
Wednesday:	11 am–7 pm
First & Third Sat.:	11 am–5 pm

"InfoTrac" (computer information) at Planetree Health Reference Center:
1. Type in "Chronic Fatigue Syndrome."
2. These categories will appear on the monitor:

Chronic Fatigue and other ailments
See also Epstein-Barr virus diseases
Chronic Fatigue Syndrome
    Bibliography
    Case Studies
    Complications
    Development & Progression
    Drug Therapy
    Evaluation
    Immunological Aspects
    Physiological Aspects
    Psychological Aspects
    Research
    Care and Treatment
    Causes of
    Demographic Aspects
    Diagnosis
    Etiology
    Great Britain
    Laws, Regulations, etc.
    Prognosis
    Reports
    Reviews of CFS Books

Key Words

For looking up information related to Chronic Fatigue Syndrome, use these words:

Adrenal insufficiency
Allergies
Anemia
Anger
Antibodies
Anxiety
Arthralgia/stiff joints
Arthritis
Autoimmune disease
Autoimmune screening (ANA)
B lymphocytes (B cells)
Candida albicans
Centers for Disease Control (CDC)
Cerebral perfusion
Chicken pox virus/
  Varicella-zoster virus
Chronic Epstein-Barr virus (CEBV)
Chronic fatigue
Chronic Fatigue and Immune
  Dysfunction Syndrome
  (CFIDS)
Chronic Fatigue Syndrome
  (CFS)
Chronic illness
Chronic Mononucleosis
Cognitive disorders
Complete Blood Count (CBC)
Cytokines
Cytomegalovirus (CMV)
Depression
Digestive function
Environmental Illness (EI)
Epstein-Barr virus (EBV)
Exercise

Fatigue
Fever
Fibromyalgia (FM)
Flu
Food allergies
Gamma globulin
Hashimoto's disease
Headaches
Heavy metal poisoning
Herpes viruses
Human Herpes Virus 6 (HHV6)
Hypoglycemia
Hypothyroidism
Icelandic disease
Immune cells
Immune system disorders
Influenza
Insomnia
Joint pain
Lethargy
Lupus
Lyme disease
Lymph glands/nodes
Magnesium
Malnutrition
Memory loss
Mineral deficiencies

Minerals
Mixed Infection Syndrome (MIS)
Mononucleosis
Multiple sclerosis (MS)
Muscle pain/weakness
Myalgic Encephalomyelitis (ME)
Natural killer cells
Parasites
Perfusion (blood flow)
Post-viral fatigue syndrome
Psychoneuroimmunology (PNI)
Retroviruses
Royal Free disease
Shingles/Varicella-zoster virus
Sinusitis, chronic
Sleep disorders/disturbances
Sore throat
Spumavirus
Stress, chronic
T lymphocytes (T cells)
Thymus
Titers
Varicella-zoster
Vitamin B-12 injections
Vitamin deficiencies
Vitamins
Yeast overgrowth

15. CFS Support Groups and Organizations

Following is a partial list of the national CFS support groups and organizations which provide support, information, referrals, newsletters. (Numbers are correct at time of publication, but may be subject to change.)

The CFIDS Association, Inc.
P. O. Box 220398
Charlotte, NC 28222
(800) 442-3437

The CFIDS Chronicle
(journal) Free information packets. Referrals and a Physicians Honor Roll.

- 35 -

CFIDS Association of Charlotte
Mr. Marc Iverson, President
P. O. Box 220398
Charlotte, NC 28222-0398

CFIDS Foundation
965 Mission Street, Suite 425
San Francisco, CA 94103
(415) 882-9986

CFIDS Treatment News newsletter available.

Community Health Services
1401 East Seventh Street
Charlotte, North Carolina 28204

Indiana CFS Support Group
810 North Bancroft
Indianapolis, Indiana 46201

Kansas City CFS Association
919 Scott Avenue
Kansas City, Kansas 66105
(913) 321-2278

Massachusetts CFSS
808 Main Street
Waltham, MA 02154

New York City CFS Support Group
845 West End Avenue, #11B
New York, NY 10025

Southern California Chronic Fatigue and Immune Dysfunction Society
3920 Market Street, Suite 115
Riverside, CA 92501

16. Self-Help Information and Organizations for Chronic Fatigue Syndrome

Working with your physician and also promoting your own healing whenever possible can help with recovery. Following are some self-help groups and organizations.

Self-Help Retreats for CFS Offered Throughout the U.S. (including Hawaii)

William Collinge, Ph.D., Director
Self-Help Retreats
2126 Green Hill Road
Sebastopol, CA 95472
(800) 745-1837
(707) 829-6813

Self-Help Retreats and Private Practice. Offices in Menlo Park and Sebastopol. Sliding-scale fee. Forthcoming book: *Recovering From CFS: A Guide To Self-Empowerment. With an Introduction by Daniel Peterson, M.D.* Putnam/Perigee. Available in summer 1993. Also, write for information on tapes available for healing, imagery, relaxation, and coping with CFS.

How To Start Your Own Support Group

The Bay Area Self-Help Center provides information and referrals, technical assistance and support, and group facilitator trainings.

Bay Area Self-Help Center
2398 Pine Street
San Francisco, CA 94115
(415) 921-4044

Free start-up packets available for forming support groups. Send name, address, phone number. Or call to order packets.

Also available: a 12-Step Directory for the San Francisco Bay Area with contact numbers for 12-Step groups—indispensible reference sources for therapists, social workers, counselors, and discharge planners, and standard reference for libraries, hospitals, social work departments, counseling centers, referral hotlines, etc.

To order a 12-Step Directory for the Bay Area: send name, address, and phone number to Bay Area Self-Help Center with a check for $10 per copy, plus $3 shipping for each copy.

Neuropsychological Information and Evaluations

Dr. Sheila Bastien
2126 Los Angeles Avenue
Berkeley, CA 94707
(510) 526-7391

For information, send a (SASE) self-stamped, addressed envelope with 45¢.

Call for an appointment for neuropsychometric testing for diagnosis of CFS and can be used for documenting disability claims.

Actualism (a meditation and healing arts school)

Actualism is a step-by-step meditation technique based upon ancient teachings, allowing you to get in touch with your divine nature. This calming yet active form of centering meditation draws upon your own resources of pure life energy and focused awareness. Its purpose is to promote health and well-being; to help you to know and fulfill your potential and purpose; and to promote mental, emotional and spiritual growth. The pure life energy is drawn upon to heal, inspire, and rejuvenate you. Actualism teaches how to gather, enlighten, and focus your awareness; and how to awaken and relate to your own inner wisdom in a wholistic process. All private or group sessions are moderately priced; fees vary according to the nature of the work. For more information, contact these Actualism Centers:

San Francisco Center
2280 Pacific Avenue #502
San Francisco, CA 94115
(415) 563-3390

New York Center
27 W. 72nd Street
New York, NY 10023
(212) 873-5826

Los Angeles Center
2762 W. Silver Lake Blvd.
Los Angeles, CA 90039
(213) 660-5283

Escondido Center
1040 S. Hale Ave., #45
Escondido, CA 92025
(619) 743-5240

Costa Mesa Center
1535 W. Baker Street
Costa Mesa, CA 92626
(714) 957-9346

San Diego Center
7484 Golfcrest
San Diego, CA 92119
(619) 462-6570

If you're not near any of the above centers call 1-800-347-2460.

Health Educational Seminars (Sponsored by J.I.C. & SelfCare Research Center)

Dr. Tom Wu, M.D., Ph.D. and Dr. Janet Wu, Ph.D., C.A.
SelfCare Research Center
P. O. Box 1111
Belmont, CA 94002-1111
(415) 591-9465

Dr. Tom Wu and Dr. Janet Wu are internationally known speakers on SELFCARE and Oriental Natural Healing programs. They combine ancient Chinese healing approaches with Western medicine. With Qi Gong, they detect early warning signs and symptoms indicating nutritional deficiencies and organ dysfunctions. They also teach preventive health care classes, including:

- Classes in building the immune system naturally to prevent diseases.
- Yin-yang concepts of life currents in relationship to health and well-being.
- Causes of disease and healing techniques to achieve balance and health.
- Nutrition and exercise programs.
- Chinese Acutechnique to relieve stress and fatigue.
- Reflexology.
- Qi Gong movements to increase Qi energy throughout the body. Any blockage of Qi may create illness. Optimal level of Qi may destroy pathogenic viruses and it may reinforce the immune system to rebalance and improve organ function, especially thyroid function. Qi may increase cellular activities, as well as improve physical appearance, mind, spirit, and relationships. Harmonizing inner and outer energy may help you to create a healthier, balanced life.

National Health Federation

The National Health Federation (NHF) is a non-profit organization which campaigns legislatively, legally, politically, and educationally for your freedom to choose whatever kind of health care you want for yourself and your family.

Call National Health Federation Toll-Free: (800) 643-4968 for information about NHF conventions held four times per year throughout the U.S.

The San Francisco Chapter meets monthly on the second Wednesday of each month and features guest speakers. For more information and for a membership application, write:

Shirley Potasz, President
National Health Federation, San Francisco Chapter
1300 Schooner, Foster City, CA 94404

17. Nutritional Supplements—Suppliers

Your doctor may suggest rebuilding your health with essential nutrients: vitamins, minerals, amino acids, fatty acids, herbs, and digestive enzymes. Some suppliers are listed below. Contact these companies for mail order catalogs and information.

The National CFIDS Buyers Club Catalog
1187 Coast Village Road, #1-28, Santa Barbara, CA 93108
Telephone: (800) 366-6056   FAX: (805) 565-3946

The Princeton Biocenter
862 Route 518, Skillman, New Jersey 08558
Telephone: (609) 924-8607   FAX: (609) 924-9423

Nutritional Enzyme Support System (NESS)
A Division of International Enzyme Foundation, Inc.
Wilmot, WI 53192

Super Blue-Green™ Algae, c/o Cell Tech. Inc.
1300 Main Street, Klamath Falls, OR 97601

MultiPlex II and Nutri-Cleanse
Lifestar International Inc., Advanced Nutritional Systems
301 Vermont St., San Francisco, CA 94103
(415) 626-6678

MultiPlex is a comprehensive multi-vitamin and mineral supplement used by doctors, nutritionists, and other health professionals in their practices. There are no synthetic or "natural source" USP or FCC grade nutrients, shellac or other animal by-products used in MultiPlex.

Nutri-Cleanse is unique among intestinal cleansers. It can be used as a bulking agent, a colon cleanser, laxative, or a meal replacement. It can even be used in baking as a source of fiber. Nutri-Cleanse is made from the finest virgin, organically grown Canadian Flax Seed.

18. Medical Test Laboratories

Your doctor may order food allergy, digestive analysis, and other tests through labs such as these listed below.

Food Allergy Laboratory

A provider of the Elisa/ACT™ (food allergy test).

Serammune Physicians Lab
1890 Preston White Drive, AMSA Blvd., Suite 200
Reston, VA 22091
Telephone: (703) 758-0610 Toll-Free: (800) 553-5472

Clinical Laboratories

Comprehensive stool tests and digestive analysis are available through this lab. Special diet and preparation of specimens are required.

Meridian Valley Clinical Laboratory
24030 - 132nd Avenue, S.E., Kent, WA 98042
Telephone: (206) 631-8922   Toll-Free: (800) 234-6825
FAX: (206) 631-8691

For depression platelet test, serotonin levels, and amino acid profile:

Min Labs, 1 (800) 831-3133 Medicare coverage

Data Test, 1 (800) 323-2784

19. Health Clinics and Community Services (such as these in the S.F. Bay Area)

Berkeley Free Clinic
2339 Durant
Berkeley, CA
(510) 548-2570

24-hour referral service
Primary medical and dental care
Psychological counseling
Appointments preferred

Berkeley Women's Health Collective
2908 Ellsworth
Berkeley, CA
(510) 843-6194

Crisis intervention and support
General medicine, gynecology
By appointment only
Open: M-F 10 am to 5 pm

Haight-Ashbury Free Clinic
558 Clayton
San Francisco, CA 94117
(415) 431-1714

Primary care
By appointment
Open: M-F 1-4 pm;
M, T, Th 6-9 pm

Lyon-Martin Women's Health Services,
1748 Market Street
San Francisco, CA
(415) 565-7667

Open: M & W 8:30 am to 8 pm
T, Th, F 8:30 am to 5 pm
No emergency care available.

Blue Oak Therapy Center
3101 Telegraph Avenue
Berkeley, CA 94705
(510) 649-9818

CFS counseling.
Jan Carlson MFCC
Reg. Intern #1MF16725
Stuart Sovatsky, Ph.D.,
Clinical Director

Buena Vista Women's Svcs.
2000 Van Ness Avenue
San Francisco, CA 94109
(415) 771-5000

Counseling Center/
Psychotherapy
Sliding-scale fee

S.F. Preventive Med. Group
645 West Portal Avenue
San Francisco, CA 94127
(415) 566-1000

Alternative/natural health care CFS specialists: Paul Lynn, MD and Denise Mark, MD. Medicare may not cover the cost.

Centers for Independent Living are located throughout California and the U.S. These organizations provide a range of services to assist people with disabilities.

Center for Independent
Living
2539 Telegraph Ave.
Berkeley, CA 94704
(510) 841-4776

Helps people with disabilities to find housing and employment, attendant referrals, benefits counseling, etc.

Center for Independence
of the Disabled, Inc.
875 O'Neill Avenue
Belmont, CA 94002
(415) 595-0783

This center in Belmont assists people with disabilities to become independent. They serve San Mateo and Santa Clara counties.

Independent Living
Resource Center
70-10th Street
San Francisco, CA 94103
(415) 863-0581

Free counseling services for people with disabilities. Attendant referrals for in-home services. Free workshops on low-cost housing.

Independent Housing Svcs.
5 Taylor Street
San Francisco, CA 94102
(415) 441-6781

Free advice regarding low-cost housing for senior citizens and for people with physical disabilities. By appointment only.

Paratransit
544 Golden Gate Avenue
San Francisco, CA 94102
(415) 202-9903

For people with disabilities who are unable to use fixed route transit, MUNI operates an extensive paratransit program—including subsidized taxi, lift van, and group van services. You need a certification form, signed by your doctor.

Department of Motor Vehicles

Disability placards available for people with CFS. You need a certification form, signed by your doctor.

20. Recommended Reading and Tapes

Following is a list of suggested books, newsletters, journals, catalogs, and tapes for healing and dealing with Chronic Fatigue Syndrome.

Books on Tape – Resources

"Braille and Talking Book Library"
Books available on tape for the disabled: (800) 952-5666. Call for an application, and return with doctor's note. Also check your local library for books available on tape.

Chronic Fatigue Syndrome Audio Tape

"Chronic Fatigue Syndrome: Information, Relaxation/Healing Exercise" by Katrina H. Berne, Ph.D. (one tape)
>Write: The CFIDS Association, Inc., Community Health Services, P.O. Box 220398, Charlotte, NC 28222-0398 ($10 per tape. Note: 6% sales tax NC residents only)

Chronic Fatigue Syndrome Books

Bell, M.D., David S. *Chronic Fatigue Immune Dysfunction Syndrome:The Disease of a Thousand Names.* New York: Pollard Publications, 1991.
>Write: Pollard Publications, P.O. Box 180, Lyndonville, N.Y. 14098. Call: (716) 765-2060.

Berne, Ph.D., Katrina H. *CFIDS Lite*. Mesa, AZ: BHB Communications, 1991.
> Write: BHB Communications, 761 East University, Suite F, Mesa, AZ 85203. ($9.50 per copy, including postage)

Berne, Ph.D., Katrina H. *Running On Empty*. BHB Communications, 1992.

Bolles, Edmund Blair. *Learning To Live With Chronic Fatigue Syndrome: Diagnosis—Zeroing in on the Real Problem; Treatment—Up-to-date Medical Help; Maintaining Physical Strength; Support Systems—Getting The Emotional Help You Need*. New York: Bantam Doubleday Dell Publishing Group, Inc., 1990.

Brooks, Barbara, and Smith, Nancy. *CFIDS: An "Owner's Manual."* Silver Spring, Maryland: 1990.
> Write: BBNS, P.O. Box 6456, Silver Spring, Maryland 20916-6456. ($19.50 per copy, including postage)

Crook, M.D., William G. *Chronic Fatigue Syndrome and the Yeast Connection*, Jackson, TN: Professional Books, 1992.
> Write: The CFIDS Assn, Inc., P.O. Box 220398, Charlotte, N.C. 28222-0398.

De Schepper, M.D., Ph.D., CA., Luc. *Peak Immunity: How to Fight EBV, Candida, Herpes Simplex and Other Immuno-Depressive Disorders and Win*. Santa Monica, CA. 1989.
> Write: Dr. Luc De Schepper, 2901 Wilshire Blvd., Suite 435, Santa Monica, CA, 90403. Or call: (213) 828-4480. ($15 per copy, $2.50 S&H, CA tax 7%.)

Feiden, Karyn. *Hope and Help for Chronic Fatigue Syndrome*. New York Prentice Hall, 1992.

Fisher, Gregg Charles. *Chronic Fatigue Syndrome: A Victim's Guide To Understanding, Treating & Coping With This Debilitating Disease*. New York: Warner Books, 1989.

Goldstein, M.D., Jay. *Chronic Fatigue Syndrome: The Struggle for Health: A Diagnostic and Treatment Guide for Patients and Their Physicians*. Beverly Hills, CA: CFS Institute, 1990.

Write: CFS Institute, 436 N. Roxbury Drive, Suite 110, Beverly Hills, CA 90210. Send: $12.95 per copy, plus sales tax 6.75%, and postage $1.50 per book.

Huggins, D.D.S., Hal. *It's All In Your Head*. Tacoma, WA: Life Sciences Press, 4th edition, 1990. (regarding mercury fillings)

Jeffreys, Toni. *The Mile-High Staircase*. Auckland, New Zealand: Hodder & Stoughton, 1982.
>   Write: Waiake Wordsmiths, P. O. Box 35 429, Browns Bay, Auckland 10, New Zealand.

Langer, M.D., Stephen with Scheer, James F. *How to Win at Weight Loss: East Well and Lose Weight Naturally*. Rochester, Vermont: Thorsons Publishers, Inc., 1987.

Lewis, Kathleen S. *Successful Living With A Chronic Illness*. Wayne, New Jersey: Avery Publishing Group Inc., 1985.

Ostrom, Neehyah. *50 Things You Should Know About the Chronic Fatigue Syndrome Epidemic*. New York: TNM, Inc., 1992.

Pitzele, Zefra. *We Are Not Alone: Learning To Live With A ChronicIllness*. New York: Workman Publishing, 1985.

Rosenbaum, M.D., Michael, and Susser, M.D., Murray. *Solving the Puzzle of Chronic Fatigue Syndrome*. Tacoma, WA: Life Sciences Press, 1992.
>   Write: Life Sciences Press, P.O. Box 1174, Tacoma, WA 98401. Call: (800) HELP-CFS to order book.

Solomon, M.D., Neil. *Sick and Tired of Being Sick and Tired*. New York: Wynwood Press, 1989.

Stoff, M.D., Jesse A. and Pellegrino, Ph.D., Charles. *Chronic Fatigue Syndrome: The Hidden Epidemic*. New York: Random House, 1988.

Wood, R.N., Terri Mosely. *Life in the Slow Lane: Coping with Chronic Fatigue Syndrome*. Madison, TN: Woodshed Press, 1989.

Chronic Fatigue Syndrome Journal

The CFIDS Chronicle: Journal of The CFIDS Association.
Write: The CFIDS Association, Inc., Community Health Services, P.O. Box 220398, Charlotte, NC 28222-0398
Phone: (704) 362-CFID (2343)   FAX: (704) 365-9755
Membership Fees: $25 per year within the U.S.

Chronic Fatigue Syndrome Newsletters

CFIDS Treatment News
Write: CFIDS Foundation, 965 Mission Street, Suite 425
San Francisco, CA 94103
Phone: (415) 882-9986   Fax: (415) 882-9758

CFS Newsletters are also available through many of the CFS Support Groups.

Chronic Fatigue Syndrome Video Tapes

"Diagnosing The Doubt: Chronic Fatigue Syndrome", CTV World Television, P. O. Box 700-820, Dept. A, Redondo Beach, CA 90277-5788 ($22.50 per video tape)

"CFS: Unravelling The Mystery" (Four-part series produced by CNN's Newsource. Limited number of copies available; $2.00 from each sale donated to fund CFIDS research.
The CFIDS Association, Inc., Community Health Services
P.O. Box 220398, Charlotte, NC 28222-0398
($12 per video tape. Note: 6% sales tax NC residents only)

Health Education Centers c/o Kaiser Permanente (HMO/Hospitals) Video tape: "Medicine in the '90s: Chronic Fatigue Syndrome–The Facts". Produced in October 1991. 57 minutes. Teleconference for Continuing Education for physicians. Note: Available to Kaiser members and to the general public.

Communication Books

Elgin, Suzette Haden. *The Gentle Art of Verbal Self Defense.* New York: Prentice-Hall, Inc., 1980.

Elgin, Suzette Haden. *More on the Gentle Art of Verbal Self-Defense*. New York: Prentice-Hall, Inc., 1983.

Smith, Ph.D., Manuel J. *When I Say No, I Feel Guilty: How to Cope–Using the Skills of Systematic Assertive Therapy*. New York: Bantam Books, 1975.

Tannen, Ph.D., Deborah. *You Just Don't Understand: Women and Men in Conversation*. New York: Ballantine Books, 1990.

Wills-Brandon, M.A., Carla. *Learning To Say No: Establishing Healthy Boundaries*. Deerfield Beach, FL: Health Communications, Inc., 1990.

Environmental Books

Center for Study of Responsive Law. *The Home Book: A Guide to Safety, Security and Savings in the Home*. Introduction by Ralph Nader. Washington, D.C., 1991.
    Write: *The Home Book*, P.O. Box 19367, Washington, D.C. 20036.

Dadd, Debra Lynn. *The Nontoxic Home & Office: Protecting Yourself and Your Family from Everyday Toxics and Health Hazards. Eliminate Indoor Pollution & Sick Building Syndrome*. New York: St. Martin's Press, 1992.

Eales, Stan. *Earthtoons: The First Book of Eco-humor*. New York: Warner Books, Inc., 1991.

EarthWorks Group. *50 Simple Things You Can Do To Save The Earth*. Berkeley, CA: EarthWorks Press, 1989.
    Write: EarthWorks Press, Box 25, 1400 Shattuck Avenue, Berkeley, CA 94709. Or call: 510-527-5811.

Ehrlich, Paul R., and Ehrlich, Anne H. *The Population Explosion: The indispensable guide to understanding and solving today's #1 environmental problem*. New York: A Touchstone Book, Simon & Schuster, 1990.

Hunter, Linda Mason. *The Healthy Home. An Attic-To-Basement Guide To Toxin-free Living*. New York: Pocket Books, 1990.

Lappé, Marc. *Chemical Deception.* Sierra Publishing, 1991.

MacEachern, Diane. *Save Our Planet: 750 Everday Ways You Can Help Clean Up The Earth.* New York: Dell Publishing, 1990.

Null, Gary. *Clearer, Cleaner, Safer, Greener: A blueprint for detoxifying your environment.* New York: Villard Books, 1990.

Rogers, M.D., Sherry A. *The E.I. Syndrome: An Rx for Environmental Illness. Are You Allergic To The 21st Century?* New York: Prestige Publ., 1986.
    Write: Prestige Publ., Box 3161, 3502 Brewerton Road, Syracuse, NY 13220.

Rousseau, David, Rea, M.D., W.J. and Enwright, Jean. *Your Home, Your Health, and Well-Being: What you can do to design or renovate your house or apartment to be free of outdoor and indoor pollution.* Vancouver, B.C.: Hartley & Marks, Ltd., 1989.
    Write: Hartley & Marks, Ltd., 3663 West Broadway, Vancouver, B.C., V6R 2B8.

Venolia, Carol. *Healing Environments: Your Guide To Indoor Well-Being.* Berkeley: Celestial Arts, 1988.

Environmental Catalogs

Eco Source: Products for a Safer, Cleaner World, "Where Quality Meets Ecology!", P.O. Box 1656, Sebastopol, CA 95473 For info.: (707) 829-7562 For orders: (800) 274-7040

The Cotton Place —Your Connection to Good Things from Nature's Fibers, P.O. Box 59721, Dallas, TX 75229, For info.: (800) 451-8866

Baubiologie Hardware, 207B Sixteenth Street, Pacific Grove, CA 93950. Call to order catalog: (408) 372-8626

Environmental Newsletters

The New Reactor, Environmental Health Network, P.O. Box 1155, Larkspur, CA 94977. Telephone: (415) 331-9804. (Dues: $10 Fixed income/disability; $25 Basic; $35 Professional)

Healthy Home & Workplace, 248 Lafayette Street, New York, N.Y. 10012. ($12 per year for four issues)

Financial Books

Phillips, Carole. *The New Money Workbook for Women*. Andover, MA: Brick House Publishing Company, 1988.

Hill, Napoleon. *Think & Grow Rich*. New York: Fawcett, 1960.

Green, Gardiner G. *How To Start & Manage Your Own Business*. New York: A Mentor Book, New American Library, 1987.

Sinetar, Marsha. *Do What You Love, The Money Will Follow: Discovering Your Right Livelihood*. New York: Paulist Press, 1987.

Slavit, Michael R. *Cure Your Money Ills: Improve Your Self Esteem through Personal Budgeting*. Saratoga, CA: R&E Publishers, 1992.

Social Security Disability Benefits Information

Brooks, Barbara, and Smith, Nancy. *CFIDS: An "Owner's Manual." Second Edition*. Silver Spring, Maryland: 1991.
    Write: BBNS, P.O. Box 6456, Silver Spring, Maryland 20916-6456.

Gentry, Jim. CFS/Disability Booklet. Graphic Imagination. Call: 1(310) 214-4653. Booklet available for $8.

Goldstein, M.D. Jay A. "Benefits Denied." *The CFIDS Chronicle: Journal of the Chronic Fatigue and Immune Dysfunction Syndrome Association*. (Spring/Summer 1990).

Ross, James W. *Social Security Disability Benefits: How To Get Them! How To Keep Them! A Guide for the Truly Disabled For The Fight of Their Lives*. Slippery Rock, PA: Ross Publishing Company, 1984.

Sindicich, J.D., D.P., *Riding The Ox Home: A PWC's (Person With Chronic Fatigue Syndrome) Guide Through The Social Security Disability Claims Process*. Corona Del Mar, CA.

Smith, Douglas M. (Attorney at Law). *Disability Workbook For Social Security Applicants.*
Write: The CFIDS Assn., Inc., P.O. Box 220398, Charlotte, NC 28222-0398

Health and Science Newsletters

University of California at Berkeley Wellness Letter, P. O. Box 420148, Palm Coast, Florida 32142. (U.S. Subscription: $24 per year for 12 issues)

Science News, 1719 North West Street, Washington D.C. 20036. New subscriptions: (800) 247-2160. (U. S. Subscription: $39.50 per year)

Health Books

Atkinson, M.D., Holly. *Women and Fatigue: Life-Changing Help For Your Personal Energy Crisis!* New York: Pocket Books, 1987.

Berger, M.D., Stuart M. *What Your Doctor Didn't Learn In Medical School: Your Guide To The Most Frequently Misdiagnosed Illnesses.* New York: Avon Books, 1989.

Brennan, Barbara Ann. *Hands of Light: A Guide to Healing Through the Human Energy Field.* New York: Bantam Books, 1988.

Carlson, Ph.D., Richard, and Shield, Benjamin (editors). *Healers on Healing.* Los Angeles: Jeremy P. Tarcher, Inc., 1989.

Chaitow, Dr. Leon. *The Body/Mind Purification Program.* New York: Fireside, Simon & Schuster, 1990.

Chopra, M.D., Deepak. *Perfect Health: The Complete Mind/Body Guide.* New York: Harmony Books, 1991.

Cooper, Ph.D., Robert K. *Health & Fitness Excellence: The Scientific Action Plan.* Boston: Houghton Mifflin Company, 1989.

Gach, Michael Reed. *Greater Energy At Your Fingertips: How To Easily Increase Your Vitality In Ten Minutes*. Berkeley: Celestial Arts, 1986.

Gawain, Shakti. *Living in the Light: A Guide to Personal and Planetary Transformation*. San Rafael, CA: New World Library, 1986.

Hay, Louise L. *The Power is Within You*. Carson, CA: Hay House, Inc., 1991.

Lidell, Lucinda, with Thomas, Sara, Cooke, Carola Beresford, and Porter, Anthony. *The Book of Massage: The Complete Step-by-Step Guide to Eastern and Western Techniques*. New York: A Fireside Book, Simon & Schuster, Inc., 1984.

Melville, Ph.D., Arabella, and Johnson, Colin. *Health Without Drugs: Alternatives to Prescription and Over-the-Counter Medicines. Including Diet, Exercise and Stress Reduction*. New York: Simon & Schuster, Inc., 1991.

Mendelsohn, M.D., Robert S. *Confessions of a Medical Heretic*. Chicago: Warner Books Edition, 1979.

Miller, M.D., Emmett E., with Lueth, Ph.D., Deborah. *Self Imagery: Creating Your Own Good Health*. Berkeley: Celestial Arts, 1978.

Ornstein, Ph.D., Robert, and Sobel, M.D., David. *Healthy Pleasures*. Menlo Park, CA: Addison-Wesley Publishing Co., Inc., 1989.

Pinckney, Callan. *Callanetics: 10 Years Younger in 10 Hours*. New York: Avon Books, 1984.

Ponder, Catherine. *The Dynamic Laws of Healing*. Marina del Rey, CA: DeVorss & Company, 1985.

Roman, Sanaya. *Living with Joy: Keys To Personal Power & Spiritual Transformation*. Tiburon, CA: H.J. Kramer, Inc. 1986.

Satchidananda. *Integral Yoga*. New York: W.H. Freeman and Henry Holt, 1987. (Gentle yoga techniques.) Call: (800) 488-5233 or (213) 886-9200.

Sinetar, Marsha. *Elegant Choices, Healing Choices: Finding Grace andWholeness in Everything We Choose.* New York: Paulist Press, 1988.

Smith Jones, Ph.D., Susan. *Choose to be Healthy: Discover how to embrace life & live fully.* Berkeley: Celestial Arts, 1987.

Siegel, M.D., Bernie S. *Love, Medicine and Miracles.* New York: Harper & Row, 1986.

Siegel, M.D., Bernie S. *Peace, Love and Healing.* New York: Harper & Row, 1989.

Stein, Diane. *The Natural Remedy Book for Women.* The Crossing Press, 1992.

UCLA School of Public Health. *50 Simple Things You Can Do To Save Your Life.* Berkeley, CA: EarthWorks Press, 1992.
Write: EarthWorks Press, 1400 Shattuck Avenue, #25, Berkeley, CA 94709.

Unity. *Daily Word.* Unity Village, MO 64065 ($5 for 1 year, $10 for 2 years.)

Weil, M.D., Andrew. *Natural Health, Natural Medicine: A Comprehensive Manual For Wellness and Self-Care.* Boston: Houghton Mifflin Company, 1990.

Creighton, M.D., Barry, Smith, R.N., Dorthy, and Young, J.D., Lise.*Understanding Laboratory Values.* Paradise, CA: Medical Resources, 1986.
Write: Medical Resources, P.O. Box 1900, Paradise, CA 95967. Call: (916) 872-8400.

Editors of Prevention Magazine Health Books. *The Doctors Book of Home Remedies: Thousands of Tips and Techniques Anyone Can Use to Heal Everyday Health Problems.* New York: Bantam Books, 1991.

Editors of Prevention Magazine Health Books. *Your Emotional Health and Well-being: How to Cope with Stress and Feel Better Fast.* Stamford, CT: Longmeadow Press, 1989.

Joklik, Wolfgang K. *Virology. Third Edition.* East Norwalk, Connecticut: Appleton-Century-Crofts. 1988.
  Write: Appleton & Lange, 25 Van Zant St., East Norwalk, CT 06855.

Health Books and Tapes – Mail Order

Contact the following companies and organizations for a current catalog of books and tapes. Note: Use postcards when writing; they are less expensive.

- (Books and tapes by Louise L. Hay)
  Hay House, Inc.
  P.O. Box 6204
  Carson, CA 90749-6204
  (800) 654-5126

- (Books and tapes by Gerald G. Jampolsky, M.D.)
  Center for Attitudinal Healing
  19 Main Street
  Tiburon, CA 94920
  (415) 435-5022

- (Tapes by John Bradshaw)
  Bradshaw Cassettes
  P. O. Box 980547
  Houston, Texas 77098
  (713) 529-9437

- (Books and tapes by Susan Smith Jones, Ph.D.)
  Health Unlimited
  P. O. Box 49396
  Los Angeles, CA 90049

- (Free catalog of books and tapes)
  New Harbinger Publications, Inc.
  5674 Shattuck Avenue
  Oakland, CA 94609
  (800) 748-6273
- R&E Publishers, Inc.
  P. O. Box 2008
  Saratoga, CA 95070
  (408) 866-6303
  (See: Order form in the back of this book)
- (Books and charts on Chronic Fatigue Syndrome)
  Pamela D. Jacobs
  750 La Playa, Suite #647
  San Francisco, CA 94121
  (See: Order form in the back of this book)

Nutrition, Herbs, and Supplements – Books

Appleton, Ph.D., Nancy. *Lick the Sugar Habit.* New York: Avery Publishing Group, Inc., 1988.

Carper, Jean. *The Food Pharmacy: Dramatic New Evidence That Food Is Your Best Medicine.* New York: Bantam Books, 1989.

Crook, M.D., William G. *The Yeast Connection: A Medical Breakthrough.* New York: Vintage Books, 1986.

Crook, M.D. William G., and Jones, R.N., Marjorie Hurt. *The Yeast Connection Cookbook. A Guide to Good Nutrition and Better Health.* Jackson, TN: Professional Books, 1989.

Dunne, Lavon J. *Nutrition Almanac. Third Edition.* New York: McGraw-Hill Publishing Company, 1990.

Hamilton, Eva May Nunnelley, Whitney, Ph.D., Eleanor Noss, and Sizer, M.S., R.D., Frances Sienkiewics. *Nutrition Concepts & Controversies.* Fifth Edition. St. Paul, MN: West Publishing Company, 1991.

Manahan, M.D., William. *Eat For Health: A Do-It-Yourself Guide for Solving Common Medical Problems*. Tiburon, CA: H.J. Kramer, Inc., 1988.

Pelton, R.Ph., Ph.D., Ross, and Pelton, Taffy Clarke. *Mind Food & Smart Pills*. New York: Doubleday, 1989.

Schwartz, M.D., George R. *In Bad Taste: The MSG Syndrome*. New York: A Signet Book, New American Library, 1990.

Tierra, C.A., N.D., Michael. *The Way of Herbs*. New York: Pocket Books, 1990.

Psychology/Self-Help Books

Bay Area Self-Help Center. *Bay Area 12-Step Directory*. San Francisco: The Bay Area Self-Help Center, 1992.
    Write: The Bay Area Self-Help Center, 2398 Pine Street, San Francisco, CA 94115. Or call: (415) 921-4044.

Beattie, Melody. *Codependent No More: How to Stop Controlling Others and Start Caring For Yourself*. San Francisco: Harper & Row Publishers, 1987.

Bradshaw, John. *Homecoming: Reclaiming and Championing Your Inner Child*. New York: Bantam Books, 1990.

Burns, M.D., David D. *Feeling Good: The New Mood Therapy*. New York: A Signet Book, New American Library, 1980.

Chopich, Ph.D., Erika J. and Paul, Ph.D., Margaret. *Healing Your Aloneness: Finding Love and Wholeness Through Your Inner Child*. San Francisco: Harper, 1990.

Copeland, Ph.D., Mary Ellen. *The Depression Workbook*. Oakland: New Harbinger Publications, Inc., 1992.

Courtney, William A. *What Works: 5 Steps to Personal Power*. Saratoga, CA: R&E Publishers, 1992.

Dinkmeyer, Ph.D., Don, and Losoncy, D.Ed., Lewis E. *The Encouragement Book: Becoming A Positive Person*. New York: Prentice Hall Press, 1980.

Gawain, Shakti. *Creative Visualization*. New York: Bantam Books, 1982.

Hall, James. *The Goal Book: Your Simple Power Guide To Reach Any Goal-& Get What You Want*. Saratoga, CA: R&E Publishers, 1992.

Helmstetter, Ph.D., Shad. *Finding The Fountain Of Youth Inside Yourself: You Can Grow Younger Every Day*. New York: Pocket Books, 1990.

Helmstetter, Ph.D., Shad. *What To Say When You Talk To Your Self: Powerful New Techniques to Program Your Potential for Success*. New York: Pocket Books, 1982.

Helmstetter, Ph.D., Shad. *The Self-Talk Solution: Take Control of Your Life—With the Self Management Program for Success!* New York: Pocket Books, 1987.

Jampolsky, M.D., Gerald G. *Out of Darkness, Into The Light: A Journey of Inner Healing*. New York: Bantam Books, 1989.

Janzen, John M. *Who Is There To Share The Dream: Finding Purpose and Potential After Tragedy*. Saratoga, CA; R&E Publishers, 1992.

Jeffers, Ph.D., Susan. *Feel the Fear and Do It Anyway*. New York: Fawcett Columbine, 1987.

Keyes, Jr. Ken. *The Power of Unconditional Love: 21 Guidelines for Beginning, Improving, and Changing Your Most Meaningful Relationships*. Coos Bay, Oregon: Love Line Books, 1990.

Lakein, Alan. *How To Get Control Of Your Time And Your Life*. New York: A Signet Book, New American Library, 1973.

Marmorstein, M.D., Jerome, and Marmorstein, Nanette. *Awakening from Depression*. Santa Barbara, CA: Woodbridge Press, 1992.

Roger, John, and McWilliams, Peter. *You Can't Afford The Luxury of a Negative Thought: A Book for People with Any Life-Threatening Illness–Including Life*. Los Angeles, CA: Prelude Press, Inc., 1991.

Rothschld, Helene, and Seff, Marsha Kay. *Free to Fly. Dare to be a Success: A personal guide to love, health & happiness.* Saratoga, CA: R&E Publishers, 1990.

Tavris, Carol. *Anger: The Misunderstood Emotion.* New York: A Touchstone Book, Simon & Schuster Inc., 1989.

Whitfield, M.D., Charles L. *Healing the Child Within: Discovery and Recovery For Adult Children of Dysfunctional Families.* Deerfield Beach, FL: Health Communication, Inc., 1989.

21. Research Funding for Chronic Fatigue Syndrome

Chronic Fatigue Syndrome is affecting millions of people worldwide. CFS is now being recognized and studied in this country. Early evidence shows that the illness causes immune system problems which can lead to many disabling symptoms. Research and education are vital to us all. Donations may be sent to the following organizations:

The CFIDS Association, Inc. is a nonprofit organization. All donations are tax deductible to the full extent allowed by law. The Association publishes *The CFIDS Chronicle* and other educational materials, provides local referrals, and directly funds CFIDS research and CFIDS advocacy efforts. The Association is governed and managed by an all volunteer board of directors comprised of people with CFS, family member, friends, and professionals.

All members receive the journal, *The CFIDS Chronicle*—the largest, most comprehensive CFIDS periodical in the United States. Membership fees are $25 within the U.S.; $35 U.S. currency for Canadian residents; and $45 U.S. currency for overseas/airmail. People with CFS may request a financial waiver if necessary. All funds contributed to The CFIDS Association, Inc. for a specific valid CFIDS purpose are so allocated. You may specify an additional contribution for research or advocacy programs. Every dollar will be spent on the targeted application.

The CFIDS Association, Inc., P. O. Box 220398, Charlotte, NC 28222 (800) 442-3437 Note: write "research" on check.

The CFIDS Foundation in San Francisco is a nonprofit organization founded in 1986 by a group of people with CFS. Funded in part by the San Francisco Department of Public Health, the San Francisco Foundation, and support from individuals, the CFIDS Foundation offers comprehensive information packets, daily telephone counseling and referrals, a Treatment Newsletter, training and materials for health professionals, patient advocacy and public policy development, media coordination, and support for research. The CFIDS Foundation accepts tax deductible donations for research. Please send check to:

The CFIDS Foundation, 965 Mission Street, Suite 425 San Francisco, CA 94103. (415) 882-9986. Note: write "research" on check.

The CFS Research Foundation is a nonprofit corporation to raise money for CFS research.

CFS Research Foundation, c/o National Jewish Center for Immunology and Respiratory Medicine, P. O. Box 6747, Denver, Colorado 80206.

Minaan, a nonprofit foundation dedicated to medical and educational matters, promotes public awareness and funding for CFS research.

Minaan, Inc., P. O. Box 582, Glenview, Illinois 60025.

SOURCES FOR GENERAL RESEARCH

Libraries

Begin your search for more information on this subject at your local library. It has a wealth of resources that you can use. Librarians are your best source of help. Ask them politely for assistance and for specific information. Also ask them for suggestions on where to look for your topic. Some of them are listed below:

Computer/CD-ROM Searches/On-Line Databases

You will find this new technology the most useful in doing any research. CD-ROM offers unlimited information for your quest.

Computer searches will give you the widest of possibilities for locating the most difficult of materials. There are many databases now available. Most larger libraries have access. You'll need to ask your librarian how to use it, but when you learn, a new world will open up to you.

Subject Guide to Books in Print
R.R. Bowker Company, New York

Over 300,000 books by American publishers are listed alphabetically in this book by subject. There are over 60,000 subject headings with over 50,000 cross references.

Subject Guide to Forthcoming Books
R.R. Bowker Company, New York

This guide lists book that will be published within the next five months.

Paperbound Books in Print
R.R. Bowker Company, New York

This book lists over 100,000 titles by subject, author and title.

Books in Print
R.R. Bowker Company, New York

This four volume guide contains over 400,000 books in print in the United States. Two volumes contain alphabetical listings by author, and two offer a listing of available books by title.

Publishers Trade List Annual
R.R. Bowker Company, New York

Here is a collection of publishers' catalogues listed alphabetically by publisher. This guide can be handy when you run across a publisher that has a number of titles on a particular subject. Using this manual can save you a lot of time if you are trying to find several books on the same subject because it lists all of the titles available from that publisher.

The Cumulative Book Index
H.H. Wilson Company, Bronx, New York

This index lists all books published from 1928 to the present that are still in print. It includes the price of each book and the publisher's address.

Director of Special Libraries and Information Centers
Gale Research, Detroit, Michigan

These three volumes have information on the collections and services of over 13,000 special collections, libraries and information centers.

World Guide to Libraries
R.R. Bowker Company, New York

If you are doing graduate work, this two volume set will help you find material that is unavailable in American Libraries. It lists over 40,000 public, university and special libraries in over 150 countries. The specialty collections often offer information that is not available anywhere else.

American Library Directory
R.R. Bowker Company, New York

If you cannot find what you want in your local library, this directory has 25,000 American and 2,000 Canadian libraries listed geographically.

Subject Collections (A guide to special book collections in libraries)
R.R. Bowker Company, New York

This important research tool lists holdings in various libraries by subject as well as special collections.

American Booktrade Directory
R.R. Bowker Company, New York

This directory contains the names and addresses of most of the publishers and booksellers in the country.

The New York Times Index–1851 to Date
Published by the New York Times, New York

Newspaper articles are also a good source of information. The Times articles are indexed by subject. In addition to providing access to articles from the premiere paper in the country, it will guide you to articles in your local paper as well.

University Microfilms, O.P. Books
Ann Arbor, Michigan

This organization has compiled tens of thousands of out-of-print books on microfilm. For a fee, they will provide a printed copy of books on demand. This service is an excellent source for hard to find works.

University Microfilms
Ann Arbor, Michigan

Dissertations and theses are an important source of original research. Ask for their Datrix Ordering Information, a kit that enables you to order a printout on any topic. The printouts are arranged by key words. You may have to supply them several key words in order to receive listings of appropriate material.

Research Centers Directory
Ann Arbor, Michigan

This directory contains information on research conducted by various colleges and universities.

Local College, University, Junior College and High School Libraries

In addition to having many of the sources listed in this guide, these educational libraries are often staffed with scholars who have expertise in your field of interest. Most of these people are generous with their knowledge.

The National Union Catalogue
Mansell, London

When this 610 volume opus is completed, it will be the ultimate source. In addition to listing the holdings of the Library of Congress, it will catalogue the holdings of the other major U.S. and Canadian libraries.

U.S. Superintendent of Documents
Washington, D.C.

Every year, the U.S. Government publishes thousands of books, pamphlets and articles on a wide range of topics. Consult your local librarian or the Superintendent of Documents to determine which libraries in your area are repositories of government publications. Many libraries have cumulative listings of the government publications.

Books for College Libraries
American Library Association, Chicago, Illinois

This listing of 50,000 scholarly titles can help you to find books that are not available in public libraries. These books may be especially useful because they are annotated.

The National Faculty Directory
Gale Research, Detroit, Michigan

Over 400,000 members of colleges, universities and junior colleges in the United States and Canada are listed in this directory. Many of them will probably be working in the area you are researching.

Union Lists of Serials in Libraries of the United States and Canada.
H.H. Wilson Company, Bronx, New York

If you are looking for magazine articles, this guide lists over 150,000 serials found in nearly 1,000 libraries. This directory can help you to obtain photocopies of the articles you want.

State Library

Your local library can borrow from the vast holdings of the state library. Most libraries maintain a union card file of the state holdings, so the chances are good they can help you find whatever book you need.

Inter-Library Loans

Most libraries participate in an inter-library loan system. If the book you want is not held at your local library, they may be able to obtain it for you from another facility.

The Center for Research Libraries
Chicago, Illinois

This excellent research center holds millions of books and microfilms. Your local library, or one near by, may be a member. If so, you may be able to borrow material from the Center.

Constance M. Winchell's Guide to Reference Books
American Library Association, Chicago, Illinois

This listing of over 8,000 reference books is the most important and comprehensive guide to reference books available.

Guide to Theses and Dissertations
Gale Research, Detroit, Michigan

This annotated, international bibliography of bibliographies will lead you to theses and dissertations from institutions of higher learning all over the world.

Ulrich's International Periodicals Directory
R.R. Bowker Company, New York

This directory that is used primarily by scholars, lists publications that are arranged by subject.

The Bibliographia Index, March 1938 to Date
H.W. Wilson Company, Bronx, New York

This semi-annual index lists large book and small magazine bibliographies.

The Reader's Guide to Periodical Literature, 1900 to Date
H.W. Wilson Company, Bronx, New York

Articles that have been published from 1900 to the present, in 160 popular magazines, are indexed in this guide. Many libraries have computerized versions of this large set of books that will make finding appropriate articles faster and easier.

Guides to Reprints
NCR/Microcard Editions, Washington, D.C.

One problem with using older bibliographies, is that many of the books listed are out-of-print from the original publishers. This guide lists tens of thousands of books that have been reprinted and are now available.

The National Archives
Washington, D.C.

The National Archives is charged with maintaining permanent records of government documents. Write to them asking specific questions regarding their holdings, and they will send you a list of items they have in your general subject area.

Library of Congress
Washington, D.C.

This source for millions of books, articles and films in all subject areas belongs to all Americans. In order to access their holdings, first check your key words against the subject headings in the Dictionary Catalogue of the Library of Congress. They use a different numbering system than most local libraries. When you get the reference number for your key word, you can use it to make inquiries for specific items. You can order a book from them on microfilm, hard copy or microcopy. Also, you can subscribe to a monthly publication of titles offered in a particular classification number. In this program, you will be sent catalog cards of new books in that number series.

Association of College and Research Libraries
American Library Association, Chicago, Illinois

This group will help you find college and research libraries in your field of interest at no charge.

Special Libraries Association
Washington, D.C.

If you are looking for libraries that have special collections on a particular topic, give this group a call.

National Directory of Addresses and Telephone Numbers
General Information, Inc.

This book lists over 200,000 addresses and phone numbers for associations, corporations and government agencies.

New York Times Index
The New York Times

You can use this index by checking under key word listings. Many libraries have this material on microfilm.

The Yellow Pages

The yellow pages for major cities can help you find specialty book stores. Your library probably has sets from around the country.

Information U.S.A.
Information U.S.A., Chevy Chase, Maryland

Mathew Lesko is an expert at discovering information sources within the U.S. Government. You may have seen him on talk shows such as Larry King Live. His company publishes a monthly newsletter that can provide you with government experts. His book, *Information U.S.A.*, published by Penguin, lists thousands of government resources.

CFS Telephone Directory

Organization	Phone Number	Page
Bay Area Self-Help Center San Francisco, CA	(415) 921-4044	37
Berkeley Free Clinic	(510) 548-2570	42
Berkeley Women's Health Collective	(510) 843-6194	42
Blue Oak Therapy Center Berkeley, CA	(510) 649-9818	42
Buena Vista Women's Services San Francisco, CA	(415) 771-5000	42
Center for Education and Mental Health San Francisco, CA	(415) 864-CEMH	43
Center for Independence of the Disabled, Inc. Belmont, CA	(415) 595-0783	43
Center for Independent Living Berkeley, CA	(510) 841-4776	43
Center for Medical Consumers (New York Library)	(212) 674-7105	29
Centers for Disease Control Atlanta, GA	(404) 332-4555	28
CFIDS Association, Inc. For recorded information: Charlotte, NC	(800) 44-CFIDS (900) 988-CFID	28 28
CFIDS Foundation San Francisco, CA	(415) 882-9986 M,T,W,Th 1-3 pm	28
Crisis Hotline for the Disabled	(800) 426-4263	29
Greater San Francisco Bay Area CFS Support Group	(510) 284-CARE	29
Haight-Ashbury Free Clinic San Francisco, CA	(415) 431-1714	42
Independent Housing Services San Francisco, CA	(415) 441-6781	43

CFS Telephone Directory (cont.)

Organization	Phone Number	Page
Independent Living Resource San Francisco, CA	(415) 863-0581	43
Indiana CFS Support Group	(317) 352-9191	29
Kansas City CFS Association	(913) 321-2278	36
Lung Line (for CFS Info.) (Mountain time)	(800) 222-5864 M-F 8am-5 pm	29
Lyon-Martin Women's Health Services San Francisco, CA	(415) 565-7667	42
Massachusetts CFIDS Assn.	(617) 893-4415	29
National CFIDS Buyers Club Catalog Santa Barbara, CA	(800) 366-6056 (805) 565-3946 FAX	40
National CFS Association Kansas City, MO	(816) 931-4777	29
National Health Federation	(800) 643-4968	40
Paratransit San Francisco, CA	(415) 202-9903	44
Planetree Health Resource Ctr. San Francisco, CA	(415) 923-3680	33
San Francisco Preventive Medical Group	(415) 566-1000	43
SelfCare Research Center Belmont, CA	(415) 591-9465	39
Self-Help Retreats Sebastopol, CA	(800) 745-1837 (707) 829-6813	37
University of California, San Francisco – Library	(415) 476-2334	33

My Personal CFS Telephone Directory

Organization or Physician　　　　　　　　**Phone Number**

My Personal CFS Telephone Directory

Support Group Leader/s   **Phone Number**

Support Group Members   **Phone Number**

(Okay to Photocopy Forms)

ORDER FORM

Books available through R&E Publishers, Inc.:

		Quantity	Unit Price
1.	*Chronic Fatigue Syndrome – How to Find Facts and Get Help* by Pamela D. Jacobs	_____	$9.95
2.	*Chronic Fatigue Syndrome – Your Wellness Workbook* by Pamela D. Jacobs	_____	$19.95
3.	*Weekly Health Care Records* (a one year set)	_____	$4.95
4.	*The Proverbs of Frank Petrini: Food For Thought* by Frank Petrini	_____	$10.95
5.	*Who is There To Share The Dream: Finding Purpose and Potential After Tragedy* by John M. Janzen	_____	9.95
6.	*Loving Bond: Companion Animals in the Helping Profession* by The Latham Foundaiton	_____	$19.95
7.	*Free To Fly: Dare To Be A Success: A Personal Guide To Love, Health & Happiness* by Helene Rothschild and Marsha Kay Seff	_____	9.95
8.	*Cure Your Money Ills: Improve Your Self Esteem through Personal Budgeting* by Michael R. Slavit	_____	7.95
9.	*What Works: 5 Steps To Personal Power* by William A. Courtney	_____	7.95

	Quantity	Unit Price
10. *The Goal Book: Your Simple Power Guide To Reach Any Goal—and Get What You Want* by James Hall	_____	6.95
11. *One Year Diet Diary: An Easy To Keep Daily Record of Your Successes* by Diane Mentzer	_____	6.95
12. *The Leadership Handbook* by Will Clark	_____	$14.95

Subtotal: $ _____

California residents add 8.25% sales tax: $ _____

Postage ($2.50 for 1st book, .50 each add'l.): $ _____

Total: $ _____

Please make check payable to:

R&E Publishers, Inc.
P. O. Box 2008, Saratoga, CA 95070
(408) 866-6303

(Please print clearly)
Ship to:

Name: _____

Street: _____

City: _____

State: _____ Zip: _____ Telephone: _____

☐ Enclosed check or money order ☐ MasterCard ☐ Visa

Card Expires _____ Signature _____